OMEGA 3 OILS

Donald Rudin, MD
Clara Felix

Avery Publishing Group
Garden City Park, New York

The medical information and procedures contained in this book are not intended as a substitute for consulting your physician. All matters regarding your physical health should be supervised by a medical professional.

Cover Design: William Gonzalez and Rudy Shur
In-House Editor: Lisa James
Typesetter: Bonnie Freid
Printer: Paragon Press, Honesdale, PA

The quotation on page 122 is from *Alternative Medicine Digest.* August 1995 Issue 7 pp. 11–12. Reprinted by permission of *Alternative Medicine Digest.*

Cataloging-in-Publication Data

Rudin, Donald O.
    Omega-3 oils : to improve mental health, fight degenerative diseases, and extend your life / Donald O. Rudin, Clara Felix.
        p. cm.
    Includes bibliographical references and index.
    ISBN 0-89529-721-3

    1. Omega-3 fatty acids. 2. Fish oils in human nutrition. I. Felix, Clara. II. Title.

RM666.O45R84 1996   615'.34
                                                                      QBI96-40090

Printed in the United States of America

10 9 8 7 6 5

CONTENTS

Preface, v

1. The Missing Nutrient, 1
2. Some Fats Are Good for You, 11
3. Our Deteriorating Diet, 25
4. How the Omega Program Developed—
   the Forty-Four-Patient Study, 39
5. Ridding Ourselves of Modern-Day
   Plagues, 51
6. The Omega Complexion Connection, 69
7. Omega Nutrition and Reproductive
   Health, 81
8. The Omega-Strong Infant and Toddler, 95
9. The Omega Way to Mental Health, 109
10. The Omega Antiaging Benefits, 127
11. The Omega Program—Phases 1 and 2, 135
12. The Omega Program—Phases 3 and 4, 151

Appendix A Sources of Omega Fatty Acids
            and Fiber, 167
Appendix B A Note to Physicians, 177
References, 187
Glossary, 201
About the Authors, 207
Index, 209

*This book is dedicated to trail-blazing orthomolecular
psychiatrist Dr. Abram Hoffer of British Columbia,
and to the memory of Dr. T. L. Cleave, Dr. Hugh M. Sinclair,
Adelle Davis, and other pioneering reform nutritionists.
Having first made us aware that modern dietary distortions
and deficiencies were intimately connected with the
unexpected and puzzling twentieth-century upsurge
in cancer, heart disease, diabetes, and mental disorders,
they then pointed the way to safe, sane,
nutritionally based solutions to these puzzles.*

PREFACE

Is it possible, in an era marked by specialization, that there could be a single, simple cure for what ails us? Our health problems abound, and we pursue each with a specially developed treatment, until one drug counteracts the effects of another and we are back where we started. But that's the very point: perhaps we should return to where we began, back to a time when we ate whole foods, fresh foods, good-for-us foods.

Of course, we can't go back in time. But we can recognize that many of the illnesses that plague us today are brought on by what we eat—or, rather, by what we *don't* eat. Modern food processing techniques have robbed our food of the nutrients we need—nutrients that we have needed since humans first walked the earth. Atherosclerosis, cancer, diabetes, obesity, immune disorders, skin problems, menstrual and fertility conditions, mental illness, and the diseases of aging are all manifestations of this imbalance.

Our bodies crave the essential fatty acids that keep them functioning properly. Specifically, they need the Omega-3 ultrapolyunsaturated oils—the nutritional missing link to a healthier life. This book examines that missing link and shows how its absence has led to what I term the modernization-disease syndrome. It also offers a simple supplement program to help you put those essential nutrients back into your diet.

The recommendations in this book result from my own pilot study in the early 1980s and from the thousands of studies that have been done since then. My forty-four-patient study provided remarkable evidence that dietary deficiencies are the basis for a host of modern-day ailments, even though individuals suffer differently from these deficiencies because of differing genetic susceptibilities. Remarkably, in a majority of cases, supplementation with Omega-3 oils brought positive results. The more formal studies conducted since then have, for the most part, borne out the original conclusions.

Chapter 1 of this book offers an overview of our modern dietary situation and looks back at two earlier diet-related diseases: beriberi and pellagra. Chapter 2 follows with an explanation of fats, the Omega-3 and Omega-6 oils, and the prostaglandins—vital substances that the body makes from the Omega fatty acids. Chapter 3 takes a hard look at our modern-day diet, and shows how our foods have gradually been robbed of essential nutrients and fiber.

Chapter 4 provides some background on my study and explains what conditions were treated with Omega-oil supplementation. Chapters 5 through 10 then show the relationships between various diseases or health problems and the absence of Omega oils in the diet. Included here are discussions of heart disease, diabetes, skin conditions, premenstrual syndrome, mental health problems, and the diseases of aging.

Chapters 11 and 12 describe in detail the Omega Program of supplementation, including information on adding vitamins and fiber to the program. Lastly, the Appendices list sources of essential fatty acids, and provide a special message to physicians regarding details of the forty-four-patient study. There is also a glossary of terms.

Sometimes it took a few months, but a significant number of the patients in my study responded in what can only be called a spectacular manner. In a few cases, responses were immediate. Omega-oil supplementation worked for them. I hope it will work for you, too.

CHAPTER 1

THE MISSING NUTRIENT

Medical research is a lot like detective work. The researcher seeks to resolve a health mystery and patiently follows leads—sometimes for years. In a novel, the mystery is solved at the end, the seemingly baffling threads of evidence woven neatly together. But medical research seldom happens that way. The evidence may be all around the researcher, but the biggest problem may be in proving that a single cause explains all of that evidence. And that is exactly the case with today's diseases.

Once, the big killers in the United States were infectious diseases. Pneumonia, tuberculosis, diphtheria, typhoid fever, and smallpox were some of the worst. But with advances in medicine, sanitation, and public health, we eliminated most of the deadly infectious epidemics. Then a series of new plagues hit us. I call these plagues modern maladies because their rates have increased along with increases in the sale and distribution of certain foods—as well as the growth of food technology—that began at the start of this century. Diabetes, cancer, heart disease, stroke, and obesity are at the top of the list, but also included are arthritis, allergies, irritable bowel syndrome, celiac disease, cystic fibrosis, anxiety and depression, hyperactivity, and schizophrenia.

What could account for such a sharp rise in these disorders? I think the answer lies, to a large extent, in the significant changes in our diet that took place at the time these diseases first started appearing in relatively large numbers of people. It started when the United States changed from a country with a largely rural population, which ate local foods, to one with a largely urban population, which relied on a national food-supply chain of highly processed foods. As food-processing techniques removed the vitamins, fiber, and other essential nutrients from our foods, the modern maladies grew rampant.

At first, nobody seemed to notice that nutrients were missing. The nutrients were essential; they were nutrients we needed in order to stay healthy. But eventually, some nutritionists and physicians realized that our diet had changed for the worse. Adelle Davis, T. L. Cleave, Denis Burkitt, Abram Hoffer, H. M. Sinclair, and many others produced research and writing that sparked a phenomenal grassroots movement. Now, people are aware of the logical connection between the foods they eat and the health problems they suffer. But there's still more to be learned.

NUTRITIONAL HISTORY REPEATS ITSELF

Before examining our nation's current dietary distortions, it is interesting to note that deficiency-caused health problems are far from a new phenomenon. Two earlier medical mysteries paralleled today's situation. These mysteries, which were eventually solved, can help us see the present health dilemma in a new light.

Beriberi

More than 100 years ago, machine-polished white rice replaced unprocessed brown rice as a staple food throughout the Orient—Japan, India, Indonesia, and most of Indochina. The reason for this change was simple: white rice keeps better. It can be stored for months or even years with little sign of deterioration. Using steel rollers, the machine-milling process scrapes off the outer husk of the rice to create a clean, white grain.

But the discarded outer husk, and the layer below it, contains most of the grain's vitamins and minerals. Without this source of nutrients, diets became deficient in thiamin (vitamin B_1). The deficiency led to epidemics of beriberi that killed and crippled thousands of people. In dry beriberi, nerves degenerate and muscles waste. Paralysis starts in the legs, and spreads over the whole body, and there may be severe psychosis. In wet beriberi, victims swell with trapped fluids and eventually suffer from congestive heart failure. The symptoms mimic those of many diseases.

Around the turn of the century, evidence began to appear that linked these mixed symptoms to one disease, beriberi, and showed that they were caused by a missing nutrient. Scientists' suspicions were confirmed by the late 1930s. Thiamin was synthesized in laboratories, and when it was introduced into the diet, many mentally ill and disease-weakened patients enjoyed miraculous recoveries. A mystery was solved.

Pellagra

The word "pellagra" is derived from the Italian word

meaning "rough skin." But pellagra affects more than just the skin. It runs a gamut of mental and physical problems. Diarrhea, dermatitis, and dementia (the "three Ds") are some of the symptoms. The mouth and tongue become bright red and ulcerated. Sometimes, the sores extend into the digestive tract, producing swelling, pain, diarrhea, and constipation. The skin may develop a scaly dryness and redden—looking wind-chapped—or become permanently scarred and thickened. Fatigue, headache, weakness, arthritis, and tinnitus—a hissing, whistling, or ringing sound in the ears—are also common physical symptoms. The mental symptoms can range from irritability, nervousness, and depression to severe neurosis and psychosis.

Pellagra had devastated Europe in the 1700s. It swept through the southern United States early in this century—ten thousand victims died there in 1915, and thousands ended up in mental institutions. The disease particularly affected poor families of sharecroppers and mill hands. Hardest hit were women of childbearing age and children between the ages of two and ten. Most of the people afflicted existed on a limited and deprived diet of refined cornmeal, corn grits, corn syrup, a little lard, corn or cottonseed oil, and white-flour biscuits. The victims seldom could afford milk, eggs, meat, or fish.

It took physicians 100 years to recognize the puzzling array of pellagra's ailments as a single disease. And even then, the nutrition connection was strongly resisted by most medical authorities, who continued to seek an infectious cause. In 1937, niacin was determined to be a member of the group of B vitamins and was identified as the long-sought "pellagra-preventing factor." Soon afterwards, medical accounts described "miraculous" recoveries, including the disappearance of psychosis, in patients given niacin. By 1941, the United States government launched a program to enrich white bread with niacin, two other B vitamins (thiamin and riboflavin), and iron. In 1945, scientists learned that small amounts of niacin could be formed in the body from the amino acid tryptophan. The corn-based diet of pellagra victims had been a poor source of tryptophan. Another mystery was solved.

THE MISSING NUTRIENT IS IDENTIFIED

Unfortunately, food-related diseases are still out there. As a researcher with thirty-five years of experience, I suspected that many modern diseases are signs of a new kind of malnutrition, an epidemic affecting America. I followed a hunch that something was missing from the average American diet—a special group of fats called the Omega-3 fatty acids. The Omega-3 fats make up one of the two families of fats, the Omega-3s and the Omega-6s, that are absolutely essential to human life. Yet the dietary availability of Omega-3 fatty acids had declined to only 20 percent of the level found in diets a century ago.

Flaxseed oil and fish oils are the best sources of these special fats, which are destroyed by modern food processing. But the Omega-3 depletion went unrecognized. Although we live in a time of nutrition consciousness, when everyone is enthusiastic about restoring nutrients to the diet, Omega-3—until recently—was virtually ignored.

I wondered what would happen if the Omega-3 fats were restored. I worked in a clinical setting, and I knew that most studies cost millions of dollars and take years to get funded and launched, so many valuable studies just never happen. Therefore, I decided to set up a small but representative pilot experiment, using volunteers suffering from chronic ailments that were not being cured by current conventional treatment. I would add the missing Omega-3 oils to their diets and see what happened.

In the two years that my forty-four-person study—which

Chapter 4 describes in detail—was underway, I witnessed dramatic changes in the people who participated. What was most exciting in this pilot study was the reduction in symptoms of many seemingly different diseases, as well as the elimination of chronic fatigue and an increase in a sense of well-being. Indeed, these have become the hallmarks of this treatment. My hunch about a missing nutrient—the Omega-3 fatty acids—had been proven correct. It was a simple experimental study, and it had worked. I had done for my patients what any good mechanic would do for your car: I changed the oil.

WHAT DO ESSENTIAL FATTY ACIDS DO FOR YOU?

Both plants and animals can make fats, using building blocks known as fatty acids. The fatty acids we humans can make are called nonessential fatty acids because we don't have to get them from the food we eat. However, there are certain fatty acids that we cannot make ourselves, but which are essential to health. These are called the essential fatty acids.

Each of the body's cells depends on the essential fatty acids for normal functioning. The cell is a tiny factory, taking in raw materials from the surrounding fluid and sending out various chemicals. Everything going into or coming out of the cell has to pass through the cell's outer surface—its membrane. The membrane depends on essential fatty acids to remain fluid and flexible. Without them, the membrane becomes stiff and unable to do its job.

Since essential fatty acids are needed by all cells, eating diets deficient in these important nutrients can result in a wide variety of disorders, including:

- Skin problems, such as itching, flaking, peeling, and hair loss

- Headache, fatigue, restlessness, confusion, and general weakness

- Easy bruising, pain, inflammation, and swelling of joints

- Infertility, spontaneous abortion, and kidney problems

Laboratory animals put on a diet lacking the essential fatty acids developed skin problems and fatty livers, were small in size and unusually susceptible to infections, and had defective reproductive systems and poorly developed brains. (For the details of one experiment, see "The Need for Fatty Acids Is Proven in the Laboratory" on page 9.) So, you can see how essential these essential fatty acids truly are.

Do we get enough essential fatty acids? I don't think we do. The average American diet is deficient in a multitude of interacting nutrients. It is also loaded with what I call antinutrients—substances that either destroy nutrients or cause nutrient requirements to soar. Although a vast quantity of food is available to people living in the industrialized world, there has been a shocking increase in diseases such as diabetes and cancer.

While these diseases are thought of as being distinct and unrelated, I believe they are actually different aspects of the new dietary deficiency disease. Just as it took more than a century for science to make the connection between B-vitamin deficiency and the diseases beriberi and pellagra, so it is taking a long time for science to acknowledge that there is a nutritional basis for the complex diseases we face today. (For more information on the problems of the modern diet, see Chapter 3.)

Why did it take so long for science to study the Omega fatty acids? The problem was a lack of equipment. A distinguished pioneer in the field, Ralph T. Holman, explains that long after scientists knew everything about the structure and functions of vitamins and amino acids, study of the essential fats was held up because the instruments needed to analyze fats in small biological samples simply didn't exist until the last quarter of the twentieth century. As there was no way to measure a deficiency of essential fatty acids in animal or human tissues, a true understanding of the powerful role played by these fatty acids in the body's regulatory systems was delayed for many, many years. However, advances in computer technology have allowed the rate of this research to soar.

Since the essential fatty acids are the main structural parts of every cell membrane in the body, we can reach a simple conclusion: a balanced intake of essential fatty acids is necessary for both healthy cell function and for the regulators that control the body's well-being. It is my belief that nutrient starvation is responsible for many—if not most—diseases today, just as it was during nutritional epidemics of centuries past. Today's public is starved for the Omega-3 oils.

INTRODUCING THE OMEGA PROGRAM

The Omega Program is based on the belief that good health is a birthright, not an accident. Like life itself, good health begins in individual cells. We all start our existence as a single-celled egg no larger than a speck of dust. Fertilized by a sperm cell, the egg divides, creating other cells, which divide again and differentiate until billions of cells form a new person. If these cells are not healthy, the whole body is not healthy.

The Omega Program is the first complete supplemental program to provide the full benefits of all essential nutrients—and their powerful interactions—when combined with a balanced diet. It is based on adding controlled amounts of Omega-3 fatty acids, vitamins, minerals, and

The Need for Fatty Acids Is Proven in the Laboratory

An important but overlooked nutrition experiment shows the need for Omega-3 fatty acids. The experiment involved monkeys—primates like ourselves with dietary needs similar to our own.

In this 1970 British experiment, eight young capuchin monkeys were placed on a laboratory diet in which corn oil was the only fat available. Corn oil—with plenty of linoleic acid, an Omega-6 fatty acid—is a standard part of the diets of laboratory rats and mice. These subprimate animals do not develop clearcut signs of fatty acid deficiency on this diet. Yet the capuchin monkeys all became sick within two years, even though their diet was supposed to satisfy every nutrient requirement.

The monkeys became very ill with a variety of problems. Two capuchins suffered long bouts of diarrhea from intestinal inflammations, and two other animals became psychotic, gnawing savagely at their own bodies, creating open, infected sores. All the monkeys developed dandruff and patchy hair loss. Four of the monkeys died. Clearly, something was very wrong.

The surviving monkeys all recovered only two months after being fed supplements of flaxseed oil, a good source of Omega-3. Thus, the tiny amount of Omega-3 in corn oil might have been enough for rats and mice, but it clearly was not enough for the monkeys—and it is not enough for human beings, either.

When human societies go on similar, Omega-3 deficient diets— diets today's nutritionists claim to be healthful—they develop the same diverse array of illnesses those monkeys did. Likewise, when modernized societies go back to traditional diets, such as during the deprivation of wartime, their modern illnesses disappear.

fiber to the diet. These substances work together to protect the body's cells from damage, which in turn can help heal or prevent a wide variety of diseases.

You should be aware that in any large group of people, there is always a chance that someone will be adversely affected by a particular food or supplement. However, the relative risk-to-benefit ratio of the Omega Program is excellent, especially if you start at government-recommended nutrient levels and work your way up to higher levels every few days. I think the real danger lies in continuing to eat the average American diet—what I call the Great American Experimental Diet because its safety has never been completely and adequately tested in primates.

In Chapters 2 through 10 of this book, you'll learn more about how essential fatty acids serve your body, and why they are important in treating specific disorders. Then, in Chapters 11 and 12, we provide a comprehensive Omega-3 supplement program, easy and relatively inexpensive to use, that you can tailor to your body's own needs.

CHAPTER 2

Some Fats Are Good for You

F at has gotten a bad reputation lately, but does it fully deserve that reputation? Many people associate fat with being overweight or obese. However, research has shown that some fats are beneficial, and that cutting all the fat out of your diet may cause you undue harm. In this chapter, I'll give you some basic facts about the different kinds of fat. Then, I'll discuss the critical role of certain fats—the Omega-3 and Omega-6 fatty acids—in the maintenance of good health. Finally, I'll explain the connection between the Omega oils we need and the foods we eat.

ALL FATS ARE NOT ALIKE

Fats, like carbohydrates, are sources of energy. The body needs fuel to function, and fats are the most concentrated source of food energy. Each gram of fat provides 9 calories, compared with only 4 calories a gram from carbohydrates.

After the body uses whatever fat it needs for energy, any excess fat does not simply disappear. It is used by many different types of tissue, but the largest amount, by far, goes to the body's adipose cells, or fat cells. These fat deposits not only store energy but also help to insulate the body and to support and protect various organs. Fats also help us absorb the fat-soluble vitamins—A, D, E, and K—by serving as carriers for them in the intestines.

The Basic Construction of Fat

All fats are made of the same basic elements—carbon, oxygen, and hydrogen. These elements are arranged in molecules called *fatty acids*. The fatty part of the fatty acid consists of carbon atoms linked together in a chain, with the acid part, which contains hydrogen and oxygen, attached to the end. There can be from four to twenty-eight carbons in the chain, so each type of fatty acid can be classified as short-, medium-, or long-chained.

But the carbon chain itself also carries hydrogen atoms. Think of a gooseneck lamp—a lamp with a long, flexible neck—with ping-pong balls attached to the neck. The lamp neck is the carbon chain, while the balls are the hydrogen atoms.

In *saturated* fats, the carbons in the chain are completely "saturated" with all the hydrogen they can carry—the lamp neck is completely covered with ping-pong balls. Saturated fats form relatively straight chains that bunch closely together. The result is a dense, solid fat, like the white fat in beef and lamb, that doesn't melt at room temperature.

In *unsaturated* fats, the carbons carry less hydrogen—the

lamp neck does not have so many ping-pong balls attached to ·+. Unsaturated fats are either monounsaturated or poly-unsaturated.

An example of a *monounsaturated* fat is oleic acid, which is found in olive and sesame oils. Each molecule of oleic acid has eighteen carbon atoms. But it does not have a full set of hydrogen atoms—two hydrogen atoms have been removed from adjacent carbon atoms in the middle of the chain. At this weakened link, the chain kinks. Because kinked chains can't bunch snugly together, fats made up of monounsaturated fatty acids are less solid and more apt to be fluid at room temperature.

Polyunsaturated fats, such as corn, soybean, and sunflower oils, are made up of fatty acids that are contain even fewer hydrogen atoms—from four to twelve fewer atoms. The fewer the hydrogen atoms, the more kinks in the chain. The more kinks, the more fluid the fat.

Special Types of Fats

Some fats, such as margarine and shortening, are created through a process called hydrogenation, in which hydrogen atoms are added to an unsaturated fat by means of high heat and metal catalysts. This process hardens the oils and gives them a longer shelf life, but destroys their essential nutritional character. Partial hydrogenation also produces "funny fats," including *trans-fatty acids*, that block the use of normal essential fatty acids.

There is another fatlike substance that you've probably heard a great deal about. *Cholesterol* is a waxy substance found in animal tissues. Most of the body's cholesterol is formed in the liver and other cells, while the rest is supplied by animal foods, such as beef, poultry, and eggs. Cholesterol is an important part of the body's cell membranes and nerve tissue.

FATS YOU CAN'T LIVE WITHOUT–
THE ESSENTIAL FATTY ACIDS

The body can make most of the fatty acids it needs from the carbon, hydrogen, and oxygen atoms provided by food. These are called *nonessential fatty acids* because it is not essential for us to consume them in the foods we eat.

However, there are polyunsaturated fatty acids that the body cannot manufacture, and these are called the *essential fatty acids*. They are necessary for good health, but we can only get them from food. There are two main groups of essential fatty acids: the *Omega-3* oils and the *Omega-6* oils. The numbers "3" and "6" refer to the place where the first kink in the carbon chain occurs. *Linoleic acid* is the primary member of the Omega-6 family, which the body can convert into the longer-chain arachidonic acid (ARA). Likewise, *alpha linolenic acid* (ALA) is the primary Omega-3, which the body can convert into eicosapentaenoic acid (EPA) and docosahexaenoic acid (DHA). Long-chain Omega-3 and Omega-6 fats form the membranes of every cell in the body, and influence every process in the cell. (See "Fats Under the Microscope" on page 16.)

The difference between the two groups is that the Omega-3 oils are more polyunsaturated than the Omega-6s. That is, the Omega-3s have fewer hydrogen atoms— and consequently, more kinks—in their molecules. This means that the Omega-3 oils are much more liquid than the Omega-6 oils at a given temperature. For these reasons, I call the Omega-3 essential fatty acids the *ultrapolyunsaturates* and refer to the Omega-6 fats as the *regular polyunsaturates*.

The production of each group of Omega oils is affected by the climate. Northern plants, in response to cold weather, produce more Omega-3 oils than Omega-6 oils. That's because the Omega-3s help to keep cell membranes fluid, permitting the membranes to function instead of freezing and fracturing. In contrast, southern plants produce very few Omega-3s but a great amount of Omega-6s. Likewise, fish in colder waters contain more Omega-3 fatty acids in their cell membranes than do fish that live in warmer waters.

Most vegetable oils we use today have high amounts of Omega-6 fatty acid, but have very little Omega-3. But the work that is done by essential fatty acids in the body cannot be done by Omega-6 oils alone—Omega-3 oils are also needed. The body works best when these two types of fatty acids are combined in the right proportions. Finding the best balance between the Omega-3 and Omega-6 fatty acids can make a big difference in total health.

FUNCTIONS OF THE OMEGA FATTY ACIDS

Why are the Omega fatty acids so important to health? There are a number of reasons. Because they form important components of cell membranes, Omega oils are needed to prevent drying and flaking of the skin. They are also needed to ensure proper growth and development in infants and children. But two of the Omega oils' most important functions involve regulating the body's use of cholesterol, and the production of substances that regulate nearly all other bodily processes.

The Omega-Cholesterol Connection

Many people think of cholesterol as being a health villain, but actually, it serves a lot of important functions within the body. Cholesterol forms a major part of the membranes that enclose every cell. As part of the cell membranes within the skin, cholesterol is changed by sunlight into

Fats Under the Microscope

When chemists talk about unsaturated fats, they talk about desaturation and double bonds. Desaturated bonds are those places in the carbon chain where hydrogen atoms have been removed. Another term for such a weakened link is double bond. The more kinks, or double bonds, a fatty acid has, the more fluid the fat will be.

In chemical notation—the shorthand chemists use to visualize how molecules are put together—polyunsaturated fats look like this:

Linoleic acid (Omega-6)

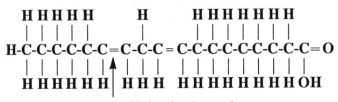

Double bond at Omega-6
position on carbon chain

Alpha linolenic acid (Omega-3)

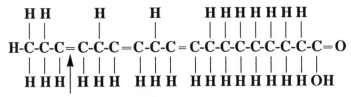

Double bond at Omega-3
position on carbon chain

C - carbon   H - hydrogen   O - oxygen

Source: D. Rudin and C. Felix, with C. Schrader, *The Omega-3 Phenomenon* (New York: Rawson Associates, 1987).

vitamin D, which regulates the body's use of calcium. It is converted in the liver into bile acids, which are needed for fat digestion. It is important for proper nerve function. It is used to create sex hormones—the chemicals that control sexual functioning. It is also used to create other hormones, such as cortisone, that control other bodily functions.

Cholesterol doesn't dissolve in water, which means it can't move through the bloodstream by itself. Therefore, the liver combines each cholesterol molecule with a long-chained essential fatty acid, and then surrounds it with protein. The resulting package, called a lipoprotein, is capable of moving through the bloodstream.

Low-density lipoprotein (LDL) carries cholesterol throughout the body for use by the body's cells. If LDL levels in the blood become too high, or if the LDLs become rancid, the cholesterol tends to stick to the walls of the arteries, which causes the arteries to become narrower. That's why LDL has been called "bad" cholesterol. On the other hand, *high-density lipoprotein* (HDL) has been called "good" cholesterol because it removes cholesterol from the blood and carries it back to the liver. Only when the diet provides enough essential fatty acids to link up with cholesterol in the liver can cholesterol do its many jobs safely.

In contrast with saturated fats, which have a tendency to increase blood-cholesterol levels, unsaturated fats lower blood cholesterol. A high blood-cholesterol level—one above 240 milligrams of cholesterol per deciliter of blood, also known as *units* of cholesterol—is considered to be a risk factor for heart disease.

Major medical emphasis has been placed on lowering cholesterol levels vigorously by means of drugs and diet. However, important large-scale studies have been done of people with high levels of blood cholesterol, and the results of these studies have been disconcerting. They show that lowering cholesterol does indeed reduce the number of deaths from heart disease over a period of years, but does not in the least improve overall mortality rates. People who achieved the lowest cholesterol levels—160 units or less—had unexpectedly high rates of death from other causes, such as liver cancer, stroke, lung disease, alcoholism, and suicide, when compared with those who had normal or high cholesterol levels.

Why would low cholesterol levels be correlated with so many serious problems? Some scientists say that very low cholesterol levels interfere with the production of crucial cell products that require cholesterol. In light of cholesterol's fundamental, nonvillainous role in the body, lowering your cholesterol level should not be the major goal. Rather, the emphasis should be on measures—dietary measures among them—that improve overall health and, as an added benefit, produce optimal cholesterol levels.

One of the dietary measures you can take is to increase the amount of Omega-3 fatty acids you consume. Omega-3 oils appear to change the balance of cholesterol in the blood—they lower the level of "bad" LDLs and raise the level of "good" HDLs.

Omega Oils and the Body's Regulators

The body also uses the Omega oils to create a variety of chemicals, called *eicosanoids*, that regulate a wide variety of bodily processes. The Omega-3 and the Omega-6 families each produce their own eicosanoids. The important role these chemicals play within the body helps to explain why the essential fatty acids are so essential.

One of the most important groups of eicosanoids is the *prostaglandins*. Medical interest in prostaglandins—extremely active biological substances made only from essential fatty acids—has grown. Prostaglandins are so vital to human life that, in 1982, the Nobel Prize in medicine went to three scientists who had studied more than a dozen prostaglandins. For purposes of simplification, the term "prostaglandin," as used in this book, may also include other eicosanoids.

Prostaglandins operate in most tissues of the body to regulate just about every bodily function, including:

- Cardiovascular and kidney system function, including dilation or constriction of blood vessels and clot formation

- Digestive system function, including regulation of stomach secretions

- The healing and repair process, including regulation of cell division

- Immune system function, including allergy responses

- The inflammatory process, including fever and pain regulation

- Nervous system function, including regulation of neural circuits in the brain

- Reproductive system function, including induction of labor or menstrual cramps

- Thermoregulation, or the maintenance of a constant body temperature

- Various other functions, including control of fluid pressure in the eyes, ears, and joints

The list seems endless—and it may be. Scientists are still discovering regulatory effects of the prostaglandins.

Prostaglandins constitute a *local tissue hormonelike system*. They work with hormones, such as insulin, that are released directly into the bloodstream and act widely throughout the body. The prostaglandins translate the directives of hormones into local instructions for local cells and tissues. In this way, prostaglandins implement hormone function on the local level, in addition to carrying out other regulatory activities.

The Omega-6 and Omega-3 fatty-acid groups each produce separate, distinct prostaglandins with different functions. For good health, both types of fatty acids are needed, and in the right ratio. That vital balance is hard to achieve because Omega-3 is often missing from the modern diet. When optimal amounts of essential fatty acids are added to the diet, many of the body's organs—including the skin, heart, kidney, liver, and reproductive organs—function better, and the body's ability to fight both cancer and infections is improved.

Exactly how do the prostaglandins work? Let's take the digestive system as an example. The efficiency of the digestive tract depends on peristaltic motion—the wavelike motion that moves food through the digestive system. The muscles that create peristaltic motion are stimulated by nerve centers called ganglia. The flow of secretions, including those that protect and soothe the digestive tract, is also induced by the ganglia. The ganglia, in turn, are regulated by prostaglandins. Therefore, digestive ailments—from gas to cramps—can be caused by prostaglandin levels that are either too high or too low.

Prostaglandin imbalances can also lead to a loss of the body's ability to protect itself. For example, certain prostaglandins in the stomach govern the secretion of a protective stomach coating that prevents digestive acids from acting on the walls of the stomach. Without this coating, the stomach would digest itself. People may be more susceptible to stomach ailments when prostaglandin imbalances cause this safeguard to fail. Such imbalances are also believed to be responsible for similar safeguard failures in other parts of the digestive system.

Supplements of Omega-3 oil can often help the body right prostaglandin imbalances. For example, a number of the patients in my study (see Chapter 4) had long suffered from digestive-system complaints, ranging from esophageal disorders to irritable bowel syndrome. Many of these patients showed substantial improvement—and, in some cases, total remission—when placed on high levels of Omega-3 supplements.

Omega Oils in Balance

Given the extensive regulatory role of the essential fatty acids, we can begin to see why dietary disruption of these fatty acids can disrupt just about any function and produce almost any disease, depending on each individual's susceptibility to specific imbalances. My work also shows a positive nutritional relationship between Omega-3 fatty acids and the amounts of fiber, selenium, and other health-promoting substances in the diet, as well as negative effects from the intake of saturated fat, trans-fatty acids, and sugar. As you'll see in later chapters, these factors all influence the production of important regulatory fats.

I must stress that the Omega-6 oils are not inherently "bad" oils—as we've seen, they are vital to human health. Rather, the problem is one of balance. Scientists speculate that our prehistoric ancestors probably ate roughly equal amounts of Omega-6 and Omega-3 essential fatty acids. Today, most people in the industrialized world eat diets with Omega-6 to Omega-3 ratios of 10-to-1 or even 30-to-1. Because of evidence that a disproportionately high intake of Omega-6 fats may be a factor in increased cancer, even conservative scientists are now suggesting that we reduce the Omega-6 fats and increase the Omega-3 fats in our diet.

For instance, in 1990, Canada's Minister of National

Health and Welfare recommended a daily 6-to-1 ratio of Omega-6 to Omega-3 fatty acids for people between the ages of twenty-five and forty-nine:

- For men (average intake 2,700 calories): 9 grams of Omega-6 to 1.5 grams of Omega-3

- For women (average intake 2,000 calories): 7 grams of Omega-6 to 1.1 grams of Omega-3

These amounts represent 3 percent of total calories coming from Omega-6 and 0.5 percent coming from Omega-3. My own estimate is that average healthy persons require no more than 6 percent of their daily calories as Omega-6 fatty acids and about 1 to 2 percent as Omega-3 fatty acids.

Sources of Omega-3 Fatty Acids

Plankton, a class of microscopic ocean plants at the base of the marine food chain, is rich in the first member of the Omega-3 family, ALA. Both fin fish and shellfish feed on the plankton and use the ALA to create the longer-chain DHA and EPA. Therefore, fish oils do not supply the simpler ALA, which the body also needs. But flaxseed yields an oil that is very high in ALA.

Flaxseed oil, and the flaxseed from which it is made, have been used in both cooking and health remedies since the days of ancient Greece and Rome. Until World War II, freshly squeezed flaxseed oil was delivered weekly to homes in northern Europe as a cooking oil. Some families have a tradition of spreading a teaspoon of flaxseed over their breakfast cereal.

Although flaxseed oil has been used for centuries, it is not as popular in the United States as are some other vegetable oils, including some—walnut, soybean, and wheat germ—that contain moderate amounts of Omega-3

ALA. However, flaxseed oil has the most ALA—50 to 60 percent. This makes it an ideal oil for cooking and for use as a diet supplement, especially if a medical condition already exists.

Flaxseed oil has some advantages over fish oil. Flaxseed oil is far more palatable than fish oil, especially when taken in large therapeutic quantities. Unlike fish oil, flaxseed oil can be used for cooking and in salad dressings, which provide easy ways to take large doses when needed. And unrefined flaxseed oil, unlike fish oil, is a source of lignan, a special kind of plant fiber that is associated with reduced incidence of breast, colon, and prostate cancers.

The body can normally use ALA to make the EPA and DHA found in fish oils. However, there are indications that some individuals cannot produce enough EPA and DHA from dietary flaxseed oil. In such cases, fish-oil supplements may be needed. Also, when flaxseed oil is the major Omega-3 in the diet of a pregnant woman, she may not be able to convert ALA into enough EPA and DHA to meet her own increased needs plus those of the fetus. Because these Omega-3 fatty acids are so important to the fetus's growth and brain development, supplements of fish oils for the mother may be necessary if she is unable or unwilling to eat seafood (see Chapter 7).

THE WAY TO BETTER HEALTH

Multiple changes in the modern diet have distorted the body's regulatory systems, producing diverse illnesses that vary from person to person, depending on each individual's genetic susceptibility. (For more information on the changes in our diet, see Chapter 3.) All this arises because the changes we've made in our dietary patterns have never been adequately tested by health authorities for their collective effects.

When our national authorities recommend eating more fish and fiber to reduce the current epidemic of heart disease, they still fail to state that:

- These recommendations are now necessary to correct a long-standing dietary deficiency of Omega-3 fatty acids, fiber, vitamins, and other essential nutrients caused by untested food refining and selection patterns.

- The benefits of supplemental cold-climate plant food oils, which are high in Omega-3 ALA, are no less important than the benefits of supplemental fish oil.

- The benefits of returning to a traditional diet are not limited to protection from heart disease, but extend to protection from all the diseases now dominating our health picture, ranging from obesity to cancer to mental illness.

Many of these diseases can be viewed collectively as an accelerated aging disease caused by diet deficiencies and distortions, similar to previous epidemics of beriberi and pellagra caused by B-vitamin deficiencies. The same food-processing and selection patterns that removed the B vitamins at an earlier time now destroy our plant and fish sources of Omega-3 fatty acids, fiber, minerals, and vitamins, all of which normally interact to produce the regulatory fats that control virtually all of our body functions.

We often hear how people who eat traditional diets have less heart disease. People in the few remaining preindustrial cultures in the world who eat traditional foods also have lower incidences of arthritis, diabetes, schizophrenia, irritable bowel syndrome—in fact, less of just about every malady that haunts the people of developed nations. The bulk of our illnesses today are not medical problems but lifestyle and nutrition problems—something you yourself can, and must, change.

CHAPTER 3

OUR
DETERIORATING DIET

I n the preceding chapters, we've seen how most
people's diets are deficient in a number of ways.
But just how did this come about? And in what
specific ways are these dietary changes causing the health
problems so many of us suffer today? This chapter takes a
closer look at the diet connection—how deficiencies in the
Omega fatty acids and fiber lead to disease, and what we
have to do to correct the problem.

THE DIET CONNECTION

Until about fifteen years ago, breast, colon, and prostate
cancers, as well as heart disease, were rare in Japan. The
traditional Japanese diet is low in both saturated fats and
hydrogenated fats. But the traditional Japanese diet is high
in fiber, and very high in Omega-3 essential fatty acids and
the mineral selenium from fatty fish such as mackerel and
salmon.

However, Japanese people living in the United States—and, increasingly, in Japan as well—are beginning to suffer from high rates of colon cancer, heart disease, and other illnesses as they adopt a modern diet. Similar situations hold true for South Sea islanders and the people of many other traditional cultures as their diets become more and more modern.

The same thing has happened to mental health. Schizophrenia, like cancer, heart disease, and diabetes, tends to appear in members of the same family. However, statistics show that all these diseases are rare in societies where traditional eating patterns include abundant amounts of fiber, minerals, vitamins, and both the Omega-6 and Omega-3 families of essential fatty acids. Even in modern societies, the incidence of these illnesses drops sharply when people abandon a diet of processed food and return to a traditional diet. Norway is a good example.

The Norwegian Notch–
A Modernized Nation Goes Traditional

The most clearly documented example of what happens when a society returns to a traditional diet occurred by chance in Norway during World War II. The incidence of schizophrenia, cancer, and heart disease had doubled in that country after 1900, when Norwegians abandoned their traditional diet in favor of processed foods. Yet, in the early 1940s, the incidence of these illnesses declined a startling 40 percent. That decline coincided exactly with the years of hardship during the German occupation of Norway.

What happened to the Norwegian diet during those terrible years? Because of the occupation, processed and refined foods were scarce, forcing the Norwegians to revert to eating traditional foods. Beans, whole grains, and fish—once staples in the diet—again became daily fare. Scientists who studied the phenomenon, which I call the Norwegian notch, found that the 40-percent decrease in schizophrenia, heart disease, and cancer coincided with a 50-percent increase in consumption of Omega-3 fatty acids. Fiber consumption probably also increased, and we know margarine consumption fell to very low levels.

After the war, the Norwegians reverted to eating commercial and processed foods. Rates of heart disease and schizophrenia soon climbed back to prewar levels.

A Food Damage Report— Nutrient Depletion in Modern Times

The Norwegian notch is only one example of the harmful effects of the modern diet. But exactly what sorts of changes have occurred in our diet over the past century? To find out, I compiled a Food Damage Report in the mid-1980s, using statistics taken from a number of sources, both governmental and private. Here is what I found:

- Consumption of Omega-3 fatty acids is down 80 percent.

- Consumption of B vitamins is estimated to be down to about 50 percent of the daily requirement. Vitamins B_1, B_2, B_3, and B_6, as well as vitamin E, have been lost in food processing.

- Consumption of fiber is down 75 to 80 percent.

- Minerals have been lost in food processing, including magnesium and chromium. Consumption of selenium, an important antioxidant, is down by more than 50 percent.

- Consumption of antinutrients—substances that hinder

the actions of nutrients—has increased substantially. Consumption of saturated fat is up 100 percent; of refined sugar, up nearly 1,000 percent; of salt, up 500 percent; and of trans-fatty acids, up 1,000 percent.

- An estimated 20 percent of today's population lives primarily on fast food, soft drinks, and alcohol.

As you can see, major changes have occurred across a broad range of diet components, not just in Omega-oil consumption. And these statistics do not even reflect the effects of chemical food additives on the diet.

The Conclusive Evidence of Food Damage

When members of traditional societies, such as the Japanese, adopt the modern diet of industrialized nations, they develop the diseases associated with modernization in short order—approximately a decade. Conversely, when members of a modern society, such as the Norwegians, revert to a traditional diet of unprocessed foods, these diseases diminish noticeably in even shorter order— within a year or two. Because of a number of studies, such as the Food Damage Report, we now know that the modern diet is lacking in a number of nutrients.

Scientific evidence of modernization's effect on our health can be drawn from experiments with monkeys who, when deprived of the Omega-3 fats, develop problems similar to our modern-day diseases. In one experiment (see page 9), a colony of capuchin monkeys developed severe deficiency symptoms when deprived of Omega-3 essential fatty acids.

More evidence came from a well-controlled 1976 study. It involved two colonies of rats, both fed identically from before conception through the time that they themselves reproduced. The only difference was that one colony was fed safflower oil, which is low in Omega-3, as the sole source of fatty acids, while the other was fed soybean oil, which is moderately high in Omega-3. It was not until the rats were adults that the safflower-fed animals showed significantly lower maze-learning ability than did the soy-fed animals. While it takes longer for subprimates to show the effects of Omega-3 deprivation, the effects do eventually make themselves apparent.

There have also been studies done with human subjects. A 1982 landmark study involved a young girl who suffered an abdominal gunshot wound that forced her to live for many months on intravenous feeding. The nutritionists supplied the usual, supposedly complete set of essential nutrients, using safflower oil as the sole source of essential fatty acids. Within two months, the girl developed a number of neurological problems: dimmed and blurred vision, staggering gait, diminished reflexes, and other conditions. Blood studies showed that the girl suffered from a marked Omega-3 deficiency. Soybean oil was then substituted for the safflower oil in her intravenous feeding. She recovered in a few weeks as her Omega-3 blood levels returned to normal.

My own study, described in Chapter 4, has also provided strong evidence of the damage done by the modern diet. Although it was but a single research project, the data that emerged indicate that some human neurological problems, as well as other systemic disorders, may well be the result of a specific Omega-3 deficiency.

THE CATASTROPHIC EFFECTS OF DIETARY MANIPULATION

How has this terrible health situation come about? There have been a number of factors. Not long after the turn of the century, when traditional diets were rapidly changing, people's intake of essential fatty acids plummeted. At that time, factory machine milling replaced local stone grinding of grains. The metal rollers produced white flour, which was inexpensive and had a long shelf life. Unfortunately, valuable vitamins, minerals, and fiber were in the grain husk and in the layer directly below the husk, which were discarded. The waste material also contained the germ, which is the embryo of the plant. The germ is a good source of vitamin E, Omega-3 and Omega-6 fatty acids, and other vitamins and minerals. But this germ was generally used for animal feed, not for human consumption.

At about the same time, with the growth of the railroads, beef could be shipped to every part of the nation. Beefsteak soon became the most popular meat. Americans had depended on local supplies of pork, fish, fowl, and game— foods relatively rich in Omega-3 and Omega-6 fats. But they soon switched to beef, a poor source of the essential fatty acids and very high in saturated fat.

Modern technology is responsible for still another loss of Omega-3 and Omega-6 fats: the solidifying of oils by hydrogenation. As we saw in Chapter 2, this involves taking a liquid, unsaturated fat and combining it with hydrogen to form a solid, saturated fat. Unfortunately, this process destroys most essential fatty acids.

Hydrogenation was developed to combat rancidity, always a big enemy of food oils, especially as part of a feeding technology on a continental scale. Reducing rancidity means eliminating or decreasing spoilage, not only in oils and shortening but in any foods prepared with them. Hydrogenating an oil extends its shelf life.

The more unsaturated, or liquid, a fat is, the more vulnerable it is to rancidity. The Omega-3 fatty acids, being the most unsaturated, are the special targets of hydrogenation because they become rancid more easily and quickly than other oils, even though the technology already exists in the food-oil industry to protect Omega-3 fats from rancidity.

The hydrogenation of food oils also creates high levels of "funny fats," known as trans-fatty acids. These artificial fatty acids behave like freeloaders, infiltrating cell membranes and stealing enzymes so that natural fatty acids can't do their work. They lodge in the muscles, liver, spleen, kidneys, adrenal glands, and heart, and appear in a nursing mother's breast milk. Trans-fatty acids actually *increase* the body's need for essential fatty acids rather than *fulfill* the body's needs. These funny fats are one of the many antinutrients in the modern diet.

By the 1950s—after a steady, fifty-year rise in the consumption of saturated and hydrogenated fats—heart attacks were epidemic. Medical research identified saturated fats in food, and cholesterol in arteries, as the prime culprits. Unsaturated fats to the rescue! Doctors using polyunsaturated oils in experiments saw lowered blood-cholesterol levels as well as lowered blood pressure in their patients. As consumers became more nutritionally aware, a penitent food-oil industry soon changed from solid, hydrogenated shortenings to liquid oils. New cooking oils and shortenings soon appeared on the market, and were supported by advertising campaigns that featured the idea of good health. Many of the new oils had a higher percentage of Omega-6 fats than before, but the Omega-3 fats were still missing.

Following the success of the new oils, margarines with higher polyunsaturated-oil contents were developed, and they were quickly endorsed by doctors and nutritionists. But the Omega-3 fatty acids in the new margarines were destroyed by light hydrogenation, a process that created even more trans-fatty acids.

In fact, calculations show that even today the net result of all these food and dietary manipulations has been to reduce the availability of the Omega-3 fatty acids in food by a whopping 80 percent compared with traditional dietary levels. At the same time, the trans-fatty acids obstruct the action of between 20 and 40 percent of the enzymes needed to utilize the essential fatty acids. Thus, the combined effect of all these nutritional distortions is equivalent to reducing dietary availability of Omega-3 fatty acids by far more than 80 percent. And this is only the beginning of the problem.

THE FIBER CONNECTION

As I found in compiling the Food Damage Report, Omega-3 oils and vitamins aren't the only nutrients that have been lost in the modern diet. Fiber has also been lost.

Fiber is the substance that gives plants structure and stability. Dietary fiber is a general term for plant materials that are not digestible. Some forms of fiber—cellulose, some hemicelluloses, and lignin—are not soluble in water, but can absorb several times their weight in water. This is called *insoluble fiber*, or roughage. It exists in the outer husk of cereal grains, and is lost when the husk is removed during the machine-milling process. Other forms of fiber—gums, mucilages, and pectin—are soluble in water. This *soluble fiber* is found in the indigestible parts of fruits and vegetables.

Fiber passes almost intact through the digestive system. Insoluble fiber provides bulk to help eliminate body wastes and helps the "good" bacteria in the lower intestine, bacteria essential to bowel health to do their job. Soluble fiber swells the food contents of the stomach and intestines, which increases the sense of fullness and prevents hunger from returning too quickly after a meal.

Natural dietary fiber not only works to keep the digestive system in order, it also acts to normalize insulin production by keeping blood sugar at appropriate levels, to prevent cancer of the bowel by binding with toxins and removing them from the system, and to help prevent other bowel diseases.

In the 1950s and 1960s, British investigators T. L. Cleave, Denis Burkitt, and others demonstrated the dietary significance of fiber. Their studies, many of them done in Africa, suggested that a lack of dietary fiber is a contributing factor in diseases of the bowel as well as in heart disease, obesity, and diabetes. Those researchers based their work on statistical evidence showing that the incidence of many illnesses increased after 1850, when machine milling of grains was introduced. These same illnesses also increase in preindustrial societies soon after they fall under the influence of modern food technology.

Machine-milling of grain destroys both essential fatty acids and fiber, and it is clear that fiber and essential fatty acids are interrelated in many bodily functions. One example is how they team up to control cholesterol levels. While the essential fatty acids control cholesterol in the blood (see Chapter 2), fiber acts to control cholesterol in the digestive tract by increasing the excretion of bile acids from the bowel. Since bile acids are made from cholesterol, existing cholesterol is then used to replace the lost bile acids. By helping to get cholesterol out of the body, fiber indirectly helps to lower cholesterol levels in the blood.

Thus, fiber and the Omega oils cooperate to normalize blood-cholesterol levels. Each can do it alone, but together they are more effective. Niacin—vitamin B3—also brings down cholesterol levels, as do exercise and weight loss. This is a prime example of nutritional synergy—different diet elements with similar effects multiplying each other's actions.

The average person's daily fiber intake in the United States is a skimpy 10 grams. Recommended intakes—

which are closer to those found in traditional diets—are from 25 to 35 grams of dietary fiber every day.

However, fiber alone does not end the problems caused by the deficiencies of the modern diet. The same is true of the addition of vitamin supplements to the diet. Supplements of nutrients such as selenium and vitamins E and C can help people recover from diseases caused by deficiencies, but vitamins and minerals alone cannot do the job.

Many of the patients in my Omega-3 study had been taking supplements for years—some in megadose amounts—and some had even added fiber to their diets. But they did not enjoy true health until Omega-3 essential fatty acids were added to the diet. Digestive ailments, along with many other chronic symptoms, respond best to supplements of fiber when the Omega-3 fatty acids are also part of the diet. Omega-3—in combination with vitamins, minerals, and fiber—is the nutritional missing link needed to ensure the efficient working of body systems.

THE SIX FACTORS THAT LEAD TO DISEASE

Unfortunately, modern dietary changes do not merely add up to produce their damage. Rather, their effects multiply because they interact together in the body to disturb the body's regulatory system. Over the decades, this modern malnutrition sets the stage for illness—the modernization-disease syndrome.

Obviously, there are a number of factors that determine how each individual is affected by these dietary changes. Let's look at some of them.

Factor 1–The Genetic Link

As physical appearance—a large nose, say, or small ears—is inherited, an increased need for certain nutrients can also be inherited, as can a susceptibility to certain diseases and conditions. A genetically weak enzyme system or an inclination toward poor absorption of certain nutrients can cause a person's dietary requirements for B vitamins, minerals, antioxidants, fiber, or essential fatty acids to be far above normal.

Genetic variations also make some people susceptible to emotional strain and other types of restless or excitable behavior. In some people even minor irritation can cause an outpouring of chemicals that raise the body's requirements for all nutrients.

When there is a nutritional deficiency, the body's regulatory system (see Chapter 2) suffers. Disease may be one result, with the same ailment striking several members of the same family because of a genetic predisposition.

Factor 2—An Essential Fatty Acid Deficiency

The Omega-3 fats are usually the ones that are deficient. This can be caused by a dietary deficiency of Omega-3, by an excessive Omega-6 intake that disturbs the balance between Omega-3 and Omega-6, or by trans-fatty acids. Any of these can block the ability of the body to use the essential fatty acids.

Factor 3—A Vitamin, Mineral, or Antioxidant Deficiency

Deficiencies in B vitamins and in minerals are common among people who get most of their carbohydrates from refined flour and sugar. A number of B vitamins are removed from refined cereal products, and are not routinely added back. This deficiency hampers the prostaglandin regulatory system because B vitamins help process dietary fatty acids into regulatory fatty acids.

There can also be a deficiency in trace minerals since they, too, are eliminated in the machine milling of grain. The minerals that are involved in the processing of essential fatty acids include—among others—magnesium, zinc, copper, selenium, and cobalt.

When deficiencies arise from a scarcity of antioxidants—namely vitamins A (and its precursor, beta-carotene), C, and E; the trace mineral selenium; and the amino acids cysteine and methionine—the essential fatty acids in body tissues become rancid and damaged. This reduces the production of regulatory fatty acids, and also produces toxic byproducts.

Factor 4—A Fiber Deficiency

Essential fatty acids and fiber work together to create healthy conditions in the bowel. They also work together to control levels of fat and cholesterol in the bloodstream. A lack of fiber creates a secondary deficiency of fatty acids by allowing the destruction of those fatty acids in the intestines. Therefore, additional essential fatty acids will be needed to counter the high blood-cholesterol levels produced by a low-fiber diet.

Factor 5—A Quietude-Exercise Deficiency

Stress—a lack of quietude in one's life—increases all nutritional requirements, including those for essential fatty acids. I saw in my pilot study (Chapter 4) that Omega-3 oils, together with fiber and vitamin-mineral supplements, increased feelings of calmness and psychological strength.

There is also good evidence from many sources that regular aerobic exercise provides important benefits to the immune system and clear psychological benefits, in addition to improving cardiovascular health. In one experiment, a group of monkeys on a high-fat diet showed less artery clogging when they were allowed to exercise aerobically for one hour three times a week over the course of a year.

Factor 6–Antinutrients and Toxic Substances

Prostaglandin formation and the use of essential fatty acids are inhibited by the following things:

- Too much saturated fat
- Trans-fatty acids
- High amounts of refined sugar and flour
- Too much caffeine and alcohol
- Smoking
- Recreational drugs
- Careless usage of prescription drugs
- Environmental pollutants

Factors such as smoking and pollutants are toxins. These toxins place added demands on the body, which in turn means that the body needs additional nutrients.

The dietary factors on the list are not really nutrients—they are antinutrients. They drain, supplant, or inhibit the actions of nutrients needed for the body's proper functioning. For example, the heating and reheating of commercial food oils—a common practice in restaurants and fast-food stores—converts some of the fatty acids to substances that may interfere with the body's ability to break up blood clots in the arteries.

HOW DO WE GET THE OMEGA-3 WE NEED?

Not all vegetable oils are alike. The Omega-6 fats have been restored via oils and margarine—often in too-great abundance—to many American diets, but most diets still lack the crucial Omega-3 oils. Moreover, the presence in our tissues of trans-fatty acids that interfere with cell membrane function requires additional Omega-3 fats just to undo that damage.

The most popular food oils are safflower, corn, sunflower, cottonseed, and peanut oils, all of which are high in Omega-6 fatty acids—but none contain more than traces of Omega-3 fats. Soybean oil, normally a good source of both Omega-3 and Omega-6, seemed to be the answer. However, because of hydrogenation and the development of a soybean with little Omega-3, it has been a nutritional disappointment.

Chemists now have the technology to reduce rancidity and still preserve essential fatty acids. I hope this technology will be used on a large scale as the public demand for Omega-3 increases.

With Omega-3 essential fatty acids stripped from our diets, do most of us get the nutrition we need? I think not. The evidence discussed in this chapter, and that uncovered by my forty-four-patient study, clearly supports that fact. Although we human beings need very little Omega-3, we aren't getting even that small amount.

How much Omega-3 oil do we need? It is impossible to say, exactly. Each person is different. Chapters 11 and 12 describe specific amounts and kinds of Omega-3 and Omega-6 oils—along with minerals, vitamins, and fiber— to be used in the Omega Program for achieving and maintaining health.

CHAPTER 4

HOW THE OMEGA
PROGRAM DEVELOPED–
THE FORTY-FOUR-
PATIENT STUDY

There have been few long-term studies of how modern changes in our diet, brought about by food-processing technologies, have affected our health. My pilot study with forty-four patients, which began in the early 1980s, was one of the few to show that one of these changes was an Omega-3 deficiency. At that time, mainstream nutritionists and doctors did not acknowledge any need for the Omega-3 fatty acids, maintaining that the Omega-6 oils were the only essential ones. Happily, there has since been a surge of medical interest in the Omega-3s, and that has fueled a great many research studies, as well as the beginning (but only a beginning!) of a turnabout in standard nutritional practice.

This chapter looks at my study in depth, with examples of how Omega-3 supplementation led to improvements in the study's volunteers—improvements that were, in some cases, dramatic enough to surprise me.

THE PATIENTS INVOLVED IN THE STUDY

I worked in a clinical setting, and my goal was to determine if the results of my pilot study would warrant a more extensive—and expensive—formal study. I wanted a certain type of patient, one who had suffered chronic complaints for more than a year, the common garden-variety complaints that take up most of the time of doctors and psychiatrists today.

There were some striking similarities in the ailments suffered by the forty-four people selected. For example:

- Ninety percent had dry-skin dermatosis—flaking of skin on the scalp, eyebrows, arms, legs, and hands, and cracking of the skin on the fingers.

- Seventy-five percent suffered fatigue, although they often didn't recognize it at the time the study started.

- Fifty percent had an immune disorder—food or airborne allergies, rheumatoid arthritis, and others.

- Forty-five percent had bursitis, tendonitis, or osteoarthritis.

- Many had headaches, itching or burning skin sensations, or tinnitus, which is a ringing in the ears.

- Many were irritable.

A number of subjects suffered many of these symptoms—and more. Other conditions included urinary-tract problems, menopausal discomfort, and irritable bowel syndrome.

I also selected patients—mostly professional people—who would not be subject to the placebo effect. That is, they would not respond with marked health improvements merely because of the special attention being paid to them as participants in a study.

I carefully noted what the volunteers had been eating at the time they entered the study. Two-thirds of them:

- Ate moderate amounts of vegetables, salads, and fruits
- Ate at least one portion of meat a day
- Ate white rice and refined flour products
- Ate bakery desserts and ice cream, and drank soft drinks
- Used butter, shortening, mayonnaise, and sugar liberally

The other third of the patients had been following the same general diet pattern, but had conscientiously adhered to a low-cholesterol diet. They used margarine instead of butter, ate lean cuts of meat, used nonfat dairy products, and used Omega-6 polyunsaturated salad oils freely. Their health was not appreciably better than that of the first group.

HOW THE STUDY WAS CONDUCTED

Initially, my patients were asked to fill out a comprehensive checklist of all their physical and mental complaints. Treatment consisted of taking individually adjusted doses of food-grade flaxseed oil or fish oil three times a day, 50 International Units (IU) of vitamin E a day as an antioxidant, and a small vitamin B supplement—two to three times the Recommended Dietary Allowance (RDA)—a day. This was in addition to any ongoing medical treatment by the patients' own physicians.

It was an informal study, in which records were kept and changes were determined by the patients' own observations, as well as by medical data and my examinations. I often cycled patients on and off the flaxseed-oil supplement, or substituted oils low in Omega-3, such as safflower and corn oils, and found that improvement varied accordingly. Therefore, a double-blind study—in which neither the patient nor the researcher knows what substance is being given—was impractical, not only because of the cost of such a study but also because taste differences among the various oils are marked.

Once a patient showed improvement while on flaxseed-oil supplements, other dietary corrections and vitamin supplements were introduced, if the patient was not already on such a program as part of earlier, conventional medical treatment.

THE RESULTS OF THE STUDY

The results of this study were impressive, as the volunteers showed improvement across a wide spectrum of conditions.

Cardiovascular Problems

Two patients who suffered angina pectoris—pain in the chest resulting from poor blood supply to the heart upon exertion—reported a complete disappearance of pain within several months after starting the flaxseed-oil regimen.

Flaxseed oil normalized one patient's high blood pressure. Two other hypertensive patients showed decreases in blood pressure, and were able to reduce their medication dosages. Conversely, one patient with abnormally low blood pressure saw her blood pressure go up to normal. This is evidence that the Omega-3 regimen can normalize blood pressure in either direction.

One woman had a varicose vein and pain in one calf that hampered her ability to walk even short distances, a condition known as intermittent claudication. She found relief by applying flaxseed oil directly to her leg, following the course of the vein. (It should be noted that some people have reported irritation or redness of the skin after applying flaxseed oil to open wounds.) Another volunteer who suffered from intermittent claudication was helped by orally administered flaxseed oil alone.

Another circulatory problem, Raynaud's disease—in which blood vessels in the hands and feet constrict abnormally, causing icy coldness—was greatly diminished in two patients.

For more information on cardiovascular problems and the Omega Program, see Chapter 5.

Emotional Problems

Nearly every volunteer reported feeling less anxious and more tranquil as they continued on the Omega Program. Some of the twelve severely mentally ill patients also showed remarkable improvement. A chronic teenage delinquent who was constantly in trouble at school and who did not respond to any other therapy—nutritional, medical, or psychological—started to behave normally six weeks after flaxseed oil was added to his nutritional supplement program.

For more information on mental health and the Omega Program, see Chapter 9.

Headaches

For years, migraine headaches accompanied the menstrual periods of one of my patients. However, the painful attacks disappeared after three months on the flaxseed-oil regimen. They recurred, in a mild form, only when the oil was withdrawn in the week before the onset of menstruation. Experimental evidence suggests that excessive production of certain irritating prostaglandins (see Chapter 2) may be responsible for migraine. The Omega-3 fatty acids tend to correct this.

Four other volunteers habitually took from two to four aspirin a day to relieve tension headaches. The headaches disappeared without aspirin several months after they began taking the flaxseed oil.

Immune Disorders

Among the study's most impressive results were those shown by volunteers with immune disorders. When the body's immune system functions improperly, an immune disease develops. The body's natural defenders, such as the white blood cells, lose their defensive powers, or even attack the body itself.

I think that a dietary deficiency of Omega-3 fatty acids is an important factor in the rise of immune disorders. Stress and deficiencies of other nutrients, such as fiber and certain vitamins, also contribute to these problems, as do inherited tendencies for specific diseases.

Half of the people in the study had some kind of immune disorder, such as food allergies, and chronic infections. A number of patients also suffered from rheumatoid arthritis, which is an immune disorder.

Many of the immune-disorder sufferers obtained relief on the flaxseed-oil regimen. Some patients saw dramatic results. One man had suffered from a hair-follicle infection in the nose for two years, even after treatment with antibiotics and steroids. This condition virtually disappeared after six weeks on flaxseed oil. And a woman who had developed a hot, swollen, and painful joint on one finger started taking two tablespoonfuls of flaxseed oil daily. Two weeks after starting the program, her problem was completely controlled.

Rheumatoid arthritis is a disease in which the immune system attacks the joints. Fluid pressure and inflammation in the joints and bursae—the sacs of fluid that lubricate joints—are regulated by prostaglandins (see Chapter 2), and certain prostaglandins can trigger inflammation. Normally, body tissues produce prostaglandins that promote a soothing internal environment. In laboratory experiments, these "good" prostaglandins have been shown to stop inflammatory arthritis in animals, the equivalent of rheumatoid arthritis in humans. The Omega-3 fatty acids keep "bad," inflammation-producing prostaglandins in check.

Of the five cases of rheumatoid arthritis treated, two severely crippled women did not respond at all. In sharp contrast, two women who had long-term cases of the disease but who were not crippled showed almost complete remission, beginning two months after the start of the study. The other woman had suffered from crippled ankles and wrists for twenty-five years, and had developed arthritis in her hip eighteen months before she entered the study. Significantly, the hip became normal, while the ankles and wrists did not.

For more information on immune disorders and the Omega Program, see Chapter 5.

Irritable Bowel Syndrome

A number of patients in the study were seeking help for digestive-system complaints, especially irritable bowel syndrome (IBS), also known as spastic colon or mucous colitis. Symptoms include abdominal pain, distension, and rumbling, and constipation or diarrhea. IBS is considered to be a functional disorder—that is, no physical cause can be found. It is triggered by many things, and is the most common disorder treated by doctors who specialize in the digestive system, accounting for about half of their practice. Many of the volunteers who suffered from IBS found some relief on the Omega Program.

Joint and Muscle Problems

Twenty of the volunteers in my study had osteoarthritis, the kind of arthritis associated with wear and tear, or the related problems of bursitis and tendonitis. Many cases were mild, and others were moderate. However, several patients were in such constant discomfort that they could not work, and in some cases required hospitalization.

I define the remission of arthritis as the disappearance of chronic fatigue, swelling, stiffness, pain, tenderness, and motion restriction. There may still be a need for a few minutes of warmup exercises on arising, as well as an occasional need for painkillers. On this basis, twelve volunteers saw significant improvement, and sometimes complete remission. In nearly all the remaining cases, there was a large drop in the consumption of aspirin and other painkillers.

Menopausal Discomfort

One volunteer reported being a cheerful, lively person at the onset of menopause eight years prior to entering the study. After menopause started, she became depressed and anxious, beset with weeping spells and the inability to think clearly. When treated with estrogen, her mood improved but she developed tender, lumpy breasts. When her doctor stopped the estrogen, her breast symptoms cleared, but her low spirits returned. The flaxseed-oil regimen permitted her to stop taking the hormone pills entirely after a few months. Her mood vastly improved, and a number of other uncomfortable symptoms—including severe hot flashes—diminished. I think that the Omega-3 corrected an imbalance in the prostaglandins that help to regulate estrogen's action within the body.

For more information on reproductive-system health and the Omega Program, see Chapter 7.

Skin Problems

Americans spend a fortune on products designed to combat dandruff and rough, dry skin. Interestingly, laboratory animals suffer dandruff and dry skin when they are fed a diet deficient in essential fatty acids. Among the patients in my study, skin problems were very common. Dandruff, dry skin, and related problems, such as sallow skin that lacked elasticity, usually cleared up within three months. Two patients had psoriasis—a disease characterized by scaly, reddish patches—and both obtained relief within four to six months after starting to take the flaxseed oil.

Other skin problems also improved. Patients who bruised easily responded to the Omega Program. Some volunteers suffered from itching, burning, or formication—the sensation of something crawling on the skin. All reported improvement after they started taking flaxseed oil. Also, even those patients who did not have overt skin problems at the time the study began reported that their complexions had improved by the time it ended.

For more information on skin conditions and the Omega Program, see Chapter 6.

Urinary-Tract Problems

One volunteer had endured the burning pain and urgency of cystitis—an inflammation of the bladder—for several years before entering the study. She reported relief two months after starting the flaxseed-oil regimen. She was still problem-free two years later.

Three middle-aged men had enlarged prostates, with difficulty and frequency in urination that had interrupted their sleep for several years. All reported that the problems disappeared after about six months on the Omega Program.

One patient was experiencing kidney problems for over a year before the study began—the passing of gritty material with blood clots in the urine. This problem was completely controlled by the flaxseed oil.

Other Benefits

I saw a variety of other conditions improve when the patients were given flaxseed oil. Several patients had taken thyroid-stimulating medications for years; they were able to stop taking such medications. Two diabetics saw their insulin requirements drop dramatically. Patients suffering from a variety of neuralgias—sharp pains that follow the course of a nerve—found that their problems cleared up after years of trouble, as did four patients who suffered from painful spasms of the esophagus. Several patients with chronic constipation and hemorrhoids also reported relief. One case of early glaucoma was helped. A number of patients were relieved of tinnitus. Many volunteers reported greater tolerance for cold weather—not surprising, since the Omega-3 fatty acids play an important part in resetting the body's "thermostat" by directing that food or stored fat be burned for heat.

Within three to four months of starting the Omega Program, a number of patients reported that they could once again drink a glass of wine or beer without feeling intoxicated and suffering the next day from a hangover. An Omega-3 deficiency may contribute to the liver's reduced ability to detoxify alcohol.

CONCLUSIONS FROM THE STUDY

The results of this study are remarkable. The flaxseed-oil supplement not only eased or eliminated the symptoms of a number of specific diseases, but it also improved the stamina, vigor, and feelings of mental well-being among the volunteers. The problems these patients had are part of what I call the modernization-disease syndrome, problems that are brought on by deficiencies related to Omega-3 in the modern diet (see Chapter 3).

My patients' health problems were not too different from the ones affecting millions of people today, many of whom are spending a lot of time and money searching for relief—without success. The Omega Program, described in detail in Chapters 11 and 12, helped my patients by providing them with the missing Omega-3 fatty acids.

CHAPTER 5

RIDDING OURSELVES OF MODERN-DAY PLAGUES

In this and the next five chapters we will take a closer look at health matters that are closely tied to the Omega oils. In this chapter, we'll see that atherosclerosis—the most thoroughly researched of the Omega-related conditions—is a complex set of problems, derived in good part from an imbalance in or lack of Omega fats. Cancer and diabetes are also problems of our modern age related to Omega-oil deficiencies, as are obesity, immune disorders, and intestinal inflammations.

ATHEROSCLEROSIS—
THE TWENTIETH-CENTURY HEART DISEASE

Heart disease was known long before this century, but it was usually related to congenital heart malformations, or to infections such as rheumatic fever. Today, people suffer

heart attacks and strokes mainly because of atherosclerosis, a buildup of plaque in their arteries that tends
to clog the arteries in the same way that waste matter clogs
a drain.

In this section, we will first look at some of the causes of
heart disease. We will then see how the Omega-3 fatty
acids can help counteract heart disease, and why standard
heart-disease treatments may not be adequate.

The Causes of Heart Disease

Why does plaque build up in our arteries? The causes are
not completely known. But we do know that cholesterol—
like butter left out of the refrigerator—can go rancid, and
that this rancid, or oxidized, cholesterol in the bloodstream
can start a dangerous chain reaction leading to a further
buildup of plaque.

As we saw in Chapter 2, low-density lipoprotein (LDL) is
the major cholesterol carrier in the bloodstream. Scientists
have always thought of it as "bad" cholesterol, the kind that
clogs arteries. But recent studies now suggest that normal
cholesterol, which serves many important functions within
the body, is not the culprit in atherosclerosis. It is only when
LDL cholesterol is oxidized that it becomes harmful. Once
oxidized, it stimulates a cascade of plaque-forming activity
in the arteries, including invasion by scavenger white blood
cells. These cells then turn into bulky, cholesterol-filled foam
cells in the developing plaque.

Apparently, cholesterol in high-density lipoprotein
(HDL) is also subject to oxidation. A high level of HDL—
the "good" lipoprotein that helps to remove cholesterol
from plaque—is associated with a greatly reduced risk of
heart disease. If oxidation occurs in HDL, its ability to
remove cholesterol from plaque foam cells is markedly
impaired.

Why does cholesterol turn rancid? Normally, a host of antioxidants—vitamins E and C, beta-carotene, selenium, and other nutrients—are carried in LDL and HDL to prevent oxidation. When dietary intake of antioxidant nutrients is low, this protection is lost. Even conservative physicians now think that ample antioxidant nutrients in food, possibly augmented by supplements, may offer the best frontline protection against oxidation of both types of cholesterol.

A heart attack usually occurs as a result of a combination of conditions, including:

- An excess of LDL carrying oxidized, or rancid, cholesterol

- A deficiency of HDL

- Platelets—the cells in the blood that promote clotting—that clump too quickly and stick to artery walls

- The formation of abnormal blood clots in the arteries

- A decrease in natural clot-dissolving factors

- Stressors that burden the heart, such as chronic high blood pressure, poor salt control in the kidneys, poor circulation, or obesity

The trigger for a heart attack is usually the formation of blood clots that adhere to an injured artery wall. These clots are especially prone to attach themselves to places that are narrowed by plaques. As these deposits accumulate, they block the flow of blood, and when major arteries of the body are involved—those serving the brain, heart, kidneys, and legs—a life-threatening problem results. Another heart-attack trigger can be a sudden spasm that squeezes the arteries, and may close down a partly blocked passage.

If a blood clot can start a heart attack, then obviously it is important for the body to protect itself against the formation of clots within the arteries. Prostaglandins, the regulatory substances discussed in Chapter 2, are important in slowing down any tendency toward accelerated blood clotting. For example, one prostaglandin called thromboxane promotes normal blood clotting; it prevents you from bleeding to death if you're wounded. Too much thromboxane, however, constricts the arteries and forces blood platelets to clump together and adhere to artery walls, which can lead to heart attack or stroke.

On the other hand, prostacyclin is a prostaglandin that keeps arteries from constricting. It also discourages platelets from sticking to artery walls unless an actual wound occurs. Hundreds of studies now show that diets rich in either fish oil or oily fish, which provide high levels of Omega-3 oils, cause thromboxane levels to fall while maintaining normal prostacyclin levels.

Heart Disease and Omega-3

Only a disturbance in the body's prostaglandin regulatory system, which depends on a proper balance of Omega fatty acids, can explain such a complex set of heart-attack triggers. For example, angina pectoris—acute chest pain caused by spasms that squeeze the coronary arteries—is related to prostaglandin-controlled spasms in other tissues, such as the spasm of the esophagus that causes choking or the spasm of the colon that causes diarrhea.

There is also evidence that prostaglandins are involved in maintaining a normal rhythm in the beating of the heart, and that Omega-3 fatty acids help prevent potentially fatal disturbances—called arrhythmias—in the heartbeat. Such arrhythmias, which cause thousands of deaths each year, can occur even when a person does not have atherosclerosis. Arrhythmia is another potential danger of having too much thromboxane in the bloodstream, since a surplus of thromboxane can promote disturbances in the heartbeat. Since Omega-3 tends to reduce thromboxane levels, it can help keep the heartbeat regular. Omega-3 can also help keep a proper amount of calcium, an important heartbeat regulator, in the heart muscle. While there is no statistical evidence that Omega-3 can help prevent arrhythmias, this is the subject of intense research.

What we've learned about the Omega-3 oils has forced science to reevaluate the connection between cholesterol and heart disease. Because cholesterol accumulates in plaque, and high blood-cholesterol levels increase the risk for heart attack, much medical research has been focused on ways to lower blood-cholesterol levels by means of medication and diet. However, given the results of some very large studies, doubt has been cast on the idea of lowering cholesterol levels as a simple way of preventing heart disease. In these studies, the people with the lowest cholesterol counts did indeed suffer fewer heart attacks, but instead died of other diseases at unexpectedly high rates. Should cholesterol reduction remain the primary goal of heart-disease treatment? I think not, because a high blood-cholesterol level is not the cause of heart disease. It is only one symptom of poor functioning within the essential fatty acid-based regulatory system. (For one example of cholesterol's often misunderstood role within the body, see "When Bad Guys Are Good Guys" on page 57.)

Traditional diets high in Omega-3 fats, such as the diet of the Greenland Eskimos (see "Fish-Eating Eskimos Suffer Fewer Heart Attacks" on page 59), apparently protect against heart disease and possibly other health problems as well. This has sparked thousands of studies on whether fish-oil fats can help everyone. Increasingly, we are seeing that complex factors—and not just high blood-cholesterol levels—affect the course of heart disease. The Omega-3 fatty acids play diverse protective roles in keeping our hearts healthy. For example, studies using fish oils that are high in the Omega-3 oils EPA and DHA show the following effects:

- Reduction in levels of thromboxane, the prostaglandin that promotes artery constriction and blood clotting

- Increase in levels of a substance, produced by the blood vessels, that helps keep the arteries relaxed and inhibits abnormal platelet clumping

- Increase in levels of clot-dissolving factors

- Inhibition of a substance that promotes the growth of muscle within artery walls, a growth that leads to plaque buildup

- Decreased production of a chemical responsible for causing the inflammation that contributes to plaque buildup

- Thinner blood, leading to improved circulation

- Increased flexibility of red blood cell membranes, which makes it easier for blood to flow through tiny capillaries

Often, the beneficial effects of Omega-3 oils produce noticeable results. For example, viscous or sludgy blood is often associated with diseased blood vessels in the feet, legs, and hands. Pain in the legs after walking a short distance—a condition called intermittent claudication—is a frequent sign of the problem. Researchers suggest that the Omega-3 fatty acids improve sludgy blood by making the red blood cell membranes more flexible, which allows the cells to travel more freely through narrowed blood

When Bad Guys Are Good Guys

Lipoproteins, the cholesterol carriers in the bloodstream, come in various types. One type, Lipoprotein (a), or Lp(a) for short, is known to be involved in arterial plaque buildup. High levels of Lp(a) indicate cardiovascular disease.

But studies suggest that Lp(a) may just be filling in for vitamin C when the vitamin is missing in a person's diet. You see, Lp(a) can take on vitamin C's antioxidant role in the blood. Lp(a) also helps a natural blood-clotting substance called fibrin lay down filaments to help repair and reinforce torn blood vessels. This can be a lifesaver when a person is bleeding badly.

So far, so good. The trouble starts when there is a chronic, long-term vitamin C deficiency. Collagen—the glue that holds blood vessels together—cannot be made without ample amounts of vitamin C. In scurvy, a disease caused by vitamin C deficiency, blood vessels actually disintegrate because there's no more collagen to strengthen them.

When there is a vitamin C deficiency, Lp(a) and fibrin work overtime trying to fill in for collagen and vitamin C. But what started out as a temporary rescue measure turns into a messy buildup of filaments in arteries. Red blood cells get entangled in the filaments, forming clots on blood vessel walls. The scene is set for the development of atherosclerosis.

Researchers say that the answer may be simple. If we keep our vitamin C levels high, Lp(a) can do its normal job and not become a troublemaker!

vessels. My treatment (see Chapter 4) of two cases of long-term intermittent claudication—and of other circulatory problems—showed remarkable results.

While most Omega-3 studies focus on fish oil, interest in ALA, a plant-based Omega-3 oil, continues to grow. As early as 1965, a study showed that flaxseed-oil supplements, which are high in the Omega-3 essential fatty acids, significantly reduced the incidence of heart disease and related deaths. And other studies show that when flaxseed oil, or flaxseed meal baked into bread, is introduced into the diet, there are beneficial changes in the blood, as well as smoother functioning of the cardiovascular system—similar in many respects to the improvements seen with increasing the amount of fish in the diet, or with fish-oil supplements. And a 1994 report in the British journal *Lancet* found that an ALA-rich diet reduced deaths from cardiovascular disease by 70 percent over a two-year period.

Alternatives to Standard Treatments for Heart Disease

Atherosclerosis often starts when one is in one's twenties, and the usual medical advice is to stop smoking, get more exercise, reduce fat in the diet, lose weight, and avoid stress. Yet the factors that burden the heart, such as chronically high blood pressure and poor circulation in small blood vessels, are controlled by the fatty acid-prostaglandin regulatory system. And this system depends on adequate Omega-3 fatty acids. Getting more exercise, not smoking, and all the rest of it is good advice, but it's not enough.

My own view is that people with certain inherited disorders may have a *greater* than average need for Omega-3 fatty acids. Their bodies may process the Omega-6 fatty acids more efficiently compared with the processing of Omega-3s. Consequently, they may require large amounts of Omega-3 fats to compete with the Omega-6 fats.

In addition, our foods and oils today routinely supply disproportionately high amounts of Omega-6 fats in relation to the Omega-3 fats (see Chapter 2). This, in itself, suppresses Omega-3 activity, creating the prostaglandin

Fish-Eating Eskimos Suffer Fewer Heart Attacks

Greenland Eskimos are responsible for some of the excitement about fish oils. In the 1960s, Danish and British scientists wondered how Eskimos could eat the highest-fat diet in the world without getting heart attacks. To find the answer, researchers trekked to remote areas of Greenland to study Eskimos who still subsisted mainly on a traditional diet of fatty fish and blubber-packed seals.

Despite their huge fat intake, the Eskimos' blood was usually neither sticky nor thick, and cholesterol and fat levels in the blood were normal. Their blood took a very long time to clot. These discoveries explained the low rate among these people of heart attacks, and the lack of blood clots in their arteries.

The fat in the fish and sea mammals that constituted a major portion of the Eskimos' diet is full of long-chain Omega-3 EPA and DHA. These fats provide these creatures with fluid cell membranes, flexible tissues, and temperature control—all advantages in Greenland's icy waters.

imbalances that bring on or aggravate illness. Nutritional treatment of heart patients shows that balanced levels of Omega-3 and Omega-6 can be beneficial in avoiding or easing heart problems.

Abundant evidence shows that heart disease is particularly affected by the powerful effects of nutrition. Since most diets are deficient in nutrients and overloaded with antinutrients, and since we tend to be overweight and to exercise too little, correcting all these interacting factors at the same time is best. In fact, there is evidence now that lowering the amount of fat in the blood through diet and exercise—and through increasing intake of the Omega-3 fatty acids—can actually reverse plaque formation. Think of it as a cholesterol flush-away.

I suspect that supplements of Omega-3 oils, in conjunction with the other health-contributing measures, flush away not only cholesterol, but also the trans-fatty acids created by modern food-oil processing, and the toxins—especially insecticides and other industrial chemicals—that pollute our environment and tend to accumulate in our tissues.

The practical effects are easy to see: fatty fin fish and shellfish, cherished in traditional diets but long excluded from diets recommended for heart patients, are real life-savers. And the same Omega-3 oils found in these foods are found in fish oils—and now in vegetarian sources (see page 61). The impact of the fish-oil studies is all the more dramatic because of the simplicity of their findings. An inexpensive nutrient has succeeded where millions of dollars spent on drugs and biomedical research have failed.

For information on how to use the Omega Program to help combat cardiovascular disease, see Chapters 11 and 12.

CANCER AND OMEGA-3

A vigorous immune system is your best defense against all kinds of cancer. The millions of cell divisions that occur daily within our bodies often produce mutants. If our immune systems did not destroy these mutants, there would be many more cancers than there are today. But cancer is still one of the major causes of death in the United States.

The Omega oils and the prostaglandins are crucial to proper functioning of the immune system. Anything that hampers this regulatory system results in a weakening of the immune system. Prostaglandins also affect the liver's efficiency in detoxifying cancer-causing substances.

Even conservative nutrition and cancer experts have acknowledged that many cancers are primarily linked to

DHA From Sea Vegetables

For people who don't or can't eat fish or shellfish, biotechnologists have extracted pure DHA, an Omega-3 fatty acid, from aquatic algae. Nonprescription vegetarian DHA in capsules is available from Martek Biosciences Corporation of Columbia, Maryland (1-800-662-6339).

dietary factors, and that breast, colon, and prostate cancers are especially correlated with high fat intake. However, research is now focused on the contrasting effects of Omega-6 and Omega-3 fatty acids on cancers. Results confirm that a high intake of Omega-6 fats increases tumor formation, size, and number. But Omega-3 fats delay the formation of tumors, and decreases the rate of growth, and the size and number, of tumors.

As we saw in Chapter 3, our diet has become deficient in both Omega-3 fatty acids and in fiber over the past century. A lack of fiber in the diet not only raises blood-cholesterol levels, but may also be an important factor in the development of colon cancer. Ample fiber dilutes any potentially cancer-causing substances in the intestines. Fiber also speeds the rate at which irritating substances travel through the digestive tract, so there is less time for these substances to affect the delicate tissue of the bowel. Generous amounts of fiber in the diet also encourage the growth of friendly bacteria in the intestines that create a climate of resistance to infections and cancer.

A fiber-generated substance called mammalian lignan has generated much research because of its exceptional promise as a deterrent to cancer. Mammalian lignan is formed in the colon by the action of colon bacteria on certain kinds of plant fiber, fiber that exists mainly in various whole grains, seeds, and berries. This fiber's job in the plant is to protect the seeds against fungi, viruses, and bacteria, and it may also do this job in the human intestines.

Breast cancer patients, as well as individuals at high risk for breast and colon cancer, have been found to make and excrete far fewer lignans than other people. Of all the high-fiber foods tested, flaxseed, either whole or ground into meal, produces the highest amount of lignans in the intestines, generating about 100 times more lignans than any other fiber source. As a result, flaxseed and flaxseed meal are being used in both animal and human studies on cancer prevention. One of flaxseed's attractions is its safety. As much as 50 grams a day, or about 5 heaping tablespoons of flaxseed meal—baked into muffins—is safe for human volunteers, even though the laxative effects for many people would preclude eating such amounts on an everyday basis. Unrefined flaxseed oil also produces substantial amounts of lignan.

Flaxseed, as we've seen, is not only a good source of fiber but an exceptionally good source of Omega-3 oils as well. A rounded tablespoon of flaxseed meal contains 2 grams of Omega-3 ALA and 0.5 gram of Omega-6 linoleic acid, as well as about 3 grams of dietary fiber. I believe that the fiber and the Omega-3 in flaxseed work together to help prevent cancer. For more information on the Omega Program, see Chapters 11 and 12.

DIABETES AND OMEGA-3

Although it was known in ancient times, diabetes has been an increasingly common problem in this century. It is now among the leading causes of death from noninfectious disease in the United States.

Two hormones produced by the pancreas—insulin and glucagon—cooperate to keep blood sugar, called glucose, at the correct level. When glucose levels are too high, the pancreas sends out insulin to force glucose from the blood-stream into the body's cells. If glucose levels are too low, glucagon sends glucose into the bloodstream for additional energy.

Diabetes occurs in two forms. The most serious form—called juvenile or Type 1 diabetes—usually strikes in childhood. It may arise from an attack by the immune system on either the insulin-producing cells of the pancreas or on the insulin receptors within the tissues. In juvenile diabetes, an essential fatty acid deficiency can cause the immune system to turn against the body instead of defending it.

The more common form—called adult-onset or Type 2 diabetes—usually appears later in life. In people who are predisposed by heredity to this form of diabetes, a diet high in sugar and fiberless carbohydrates can eventually stress the insulin production mechanism. Hypoglycemia, or low blood sugar, may represent an early phase of diabetes, in which a hair-trigger response from the over-worked pancreas sends out too much insulin. Eventually, the body stops responding to the pancreas's signals, and blood levels of both insulin and sugar go up.

As we've seen, all hormones, including insulin and glucagon, exert their control over the cells by stimulating production of local regulatory chemicals called prostaglandins. In turn, the prostaglandins pass the message of the hormones to the individual cells. The prostaglandins are made from essential fatty acids. Therefore, a deficiency of essential fatty acids, or of the vitamins or minerals they need to be effective, interferes with prostaglandin production. This can intensify adult-onset diabetes even though adequate insulin is produced.

The essential fatty acids also affect the ability of the body's cells to respond to insulin. In a 1993 study, Australian researchers learned that insulin resistance is related to what kinds of fatty acids make up the cell membranes. The more

Omega-3 and Omega-6 fatty acids there are in the cell membranes of adult diabetics, the more their tissues respond to insulin.

Some diabetics seem to be blocked from converting short-chain Omega-6 linoleic acid into the longer-chain acids needed for both cell membranes and prostaglandins (see Chapter 2). Noted researcher David Horrobin and others are using supplements of evening primrose oil, which contains an Omega-6 oil called gamma linolenic acid (GLA), to bypass the blocked processes. Damage to nerves, a big problem for many diabetic persons, has been halted or even reversed by GLA supplements.

Degeneration of the eye's retina—the projection screen on which light that passes through the eye is thrown—is a common cause of blindness in severe cases of diabetes. An Omega-3 oil called DHA is the most abundant polyunsaturated fat in the retina, an oil that is normally made by the body from the basic Omega-3 oil, ALA. However, the high blood-sugar levels seen in diabetes block the conversion of ALA into DHA. The block may be partly overcome by eating foods, mainly fatty fish, that contain ample amounts of ready-made DHA.

As we've seen in the case of cancer, studies now indicate that dietary fiber can help to prevent diabetes or to affect its course by reducing insulin requirements. I think Omega-3 supplements can do the same thing. A fiber deficiency, coupled with an Omega-3 deficiency, magnifies all the blood-sugar problems seen in diabetes. Normally, fiber acts as a buffer in the digestive tract by slowing the release of sugar into the bloodstream. Without fiber, the refined starches and sugars in processed foods quickly create a big surge of glucose and a never-ending demand for insulin.

Fiber is an important component of the Omega Program. For information on how to use the program to fight diabetes, see Chapters 11 and 12.

OTHER DISEASES AND OMEGA-3

While a lot of Omega-3 research has concentrated on major diseases, such as heart disease and cancer, the Omega-3 fatty acids have been shown to be important in curbing various other afflictions.

Obesity

Obesity is a serious disorder of modern times. Compared with other people, the obese—people who are more than 20 percent over normal weight—tend to have a host of health problems, including:

- High blood pressure

- Elevated blood-cholesterol levels

- Adult-onset diabetes

- Cancer—of the colon, rectum, and prostate in men, and of the breast, uterus, ovaries, and cervix in women

There is more to eliminating obesity than merely reducing one's weight. Obesity is just one more disease of modernization, caused by a deficiency of essential fatty acids and other vital nutrients, combined with a surplus of antinutrients. This modernization-disease syndrome can attack the appetite-controlling mechanism in the brain, as well as the body's heat-controlling, calorie-burning system. As a result, you take in more calories than you burn off. The resultant weight gain has been properly called "no-fault fat"—willpower has nothing to do with it.

Once obesity becomes a problem, it compounds other stresses or genetic weak spots. The high levels of insulin and fat in the bloodstream that often develop in the obese individual can aggravate heart disease and diabetes.

To overcome obesity, a person must exercise properly and switch to a diet that provides Omega-3 fatty acids, fiber, and all the other required nutrients, and that reduces the amounts of antinutrients such as sugar and saturated fats. The Omega Program, which can help fight obesity, is described in Chapters 11 and 12.

Immune Disorders

Immune disorders are rampant in modern societies. As we saw in Chapter 4, they cover a huge range of illnesses, from rheumatoid arthritis to allergies. And as we noted earlier, both cancer and juvenile diabetes involve some element of immune disorder. Immune disorders generally develop when the body's system of defense against foreign invaders goes out of control and starts attacking the body itself.

Normally, the immune system is kept under control by the body's essential fatty acid-based regulatory system. But dietary distortions, especially a shortage of the Omega-3 fatty acids, are now known to contribute to—or even prompt—the breakdown of the immune system. Harumi Okuyama, a Japanese scientist, reports that he has seen a significant rise in the rate of allergies among Japanese babies—one-third of the infants born in Japan are now diagnosed with allergic disorders. He attributes this increase to Westernized changes in the Japanese diet. He says that reduced Omega-3 intake, coupled with excessive Omega-6 intake, leads to overproduction of irritating Omega-6 prostaglandins.

I am convinced that the way to reduce immune disorders is to bring the intake of Omega-3 and Omega-6 fatty acids into balance, mainly by increasing Omega-3 intake to counteract excessive Omega-6 intake. For information on the Omega Program, see Chapters 11 and 12.

Chronic Intestinal Inflammation

More and more people in their twenties are coming down with Crohn's disease, which is characterized by diarrhea, abdominal pain, fever, weight loss, and weakness. These symptoms stem from an inflammation of the small intestine, and sometimes of the large intestine as well. While the ailment tends to be chronic, patients may have long disease-free periods, known as remissions, between flare-ups.

In one study, doctors in Bologna and Turin, Italy, gave fish-oil capsules three times a day for one year to thirty-nine Crohn's patients who had been in remission for about eight months. A similar control group of thirty-nine patients received capsules that contained neutral oils. The fish-oil capsules were specially formulated to reduce fishy odor and to improve absorption of Omega-3 EPA and DHA. Reducing the odor was important, because until the trial was over, neither the doctors nor the patients knew which patients had gotten which oils. After a year of ingesting 2.7 grams of EPA and DHA every day, twenty-three of the patients who received the fish oils were still in remission. By contrast, only eleven of the thirty-nine control patients stayed in remission.

In Crohn's disease, bowel tissue contains abnormally high levels of inflammation-producing, "bad" prostaglandins from Omega-6 ARA. In the patients taking the fish oil whose illness remained in remission, red blood cell levels of ARA plunged, while levels of Omega-3 EPA and DHA rose greatly. In general, laboratory tests indicated that inflammation decreased in the fish-oil patients, but increased in the control patients.

Ulcerative colitis is another chronic inflammatory disease, usually of the large intestine, in which ulceration and erosion of the bowel tissue cause severe diarrhea and loss of blood, as well as weakness and weight loss.

As in Crohn's disease, bowel tissue shows high levels of "bad," ARA-produced prostaglandins. The worse the symptoms, the higher the levels of these trouble-making prostaglandins. In one study, conducted by William Stenson of Washington University School of Medicine, twenty-four patients with active ulcerative colitis who took fish-oil capsules for four months showed a big drop in "bad" prostaglandins. These patients also showed bowel tissue healing and reduced rectal bleeding, and they gained badly needed weight. The capsules contained 5.4 grams of EPA and DHA. Moreover, seven patients who were also getting prednisone, a steroid drug, were able to cut their dosages in half.

THE DISEASE-REDUCING POTENTIAL OF OMEGA-3

Since I began to study Omega-3 deficiencies in the early 1980s, research in this field has seen an exponential surge. Between 1985 and 1993, close to 5,000 medical studies on Omega-3 fatty acids emerged worldwide. If anything, the pace has quickened since then, as more and more optimistic reports on Omega-3 benefits in terms of heart disease and other ailments are confirmed.

The original focus of these studies was on the cardiovascular system, but it soon expanded to include studies on cancer, arthritis, psoriasis, and various inflammatory and immune disorders, including kidney disease. Though the emphasis remains on heart disease—the major killer in industrialized countries such as the United States—it is becoming evident that many of these conditions are a result of modernization, and that balancing the essential fatty acids in our diet will rid us of some of the diseases that plague our modern world.

CHAPTER 6

THE OMEGA
COMPLEXION
CONNECTION

B eautiful complexions come in every shade, from creamy ivory and pinky peach to burnished black and glowing copper. At any age, smooth, velvety, unbroken, luminescent skin is lovely to look at and signals good health.

However, lovely skin often evades us. Each year, people in the United States spend more than $10 billion on over-the-counter skin preparations and medical treatments. And while some people simply want to appear more youthful, there are skin conditions that can involve extreme discomfort, even disfigurement. In this chapter, we'll explore the connection between good nutrition and good skin, and we'll see why the Omega-3 fatty acids are so important to your skin's health.

WHAT YOUR SKIN DOES FOR YOU

Skin is a protective wrapping. Besides packaging the outside of your body, skin protects your body by guarding it against the ultraviolet rays of the sun, traumas such as bangs and cuts, and invasions by bacteria. Skin also shields you from environmental attacks, such as those that come from pollution.

Your skin is the largest organ of your body—an average person's skin covers about 19 square feet in area. Skin varies in thickness from 0.2 millimeters to 0.3 millimeters—thinner than a hair—on the eyelids, to about 4 millimeters on the back and shoulders. The skin on the soles of the feet is the thickest of all.

There are two main layers to the skin—the upper layer, or epidermis, and the lower layer, or dermis. The epidermis is made up of several cell layers. It is formed through the activity of the basal layer, a single layer of cells at the bottom of the epidermis. These cells constantly divide, creating new cells. New cells migrate from the basal layer to the skin's surface in about three or four weeks. As you age, the migration slows, and the same cells remain on your skin's surface longer and longer. These older, less efficient cells lose moisture and elasticity, resulting in a dry, slack surface. The epidermis also contains the cells that give skin its color.

The dermis is divided into two layers and is made up of connective tissue. It contains blood and lymph vessels, as well as nerve endings, hair follicles, sweat glands, and sebaceous glands, which produce the skin's oils. This immense network of blood and lymph vessels brings nutrients to the skin and removes waste. The skin is made up of about 70 percent water, 27 percent protein, 2 percent fat, and 1 percent sugar. The oils in the skin include both essential and nonessential fatty acids, and fatty substances such as cholesterol, all of which keep the skin smooth and glossy.

Under the dermis, the hypodermis, also known as the subcutaneous tissue, connects the skin to the underlying muscles and is made of loose connective tissue. It also serves as a fat-storage and insulation layer. The hair follicles are rooted in the hypodermis, as are many of the sweat glands. Hair follicles—tiny, well-like pores—send hair out to the surface of the skin.

Nail is also a specialized form of skin, related to the horns, hoofs, and claws of animals and birds. The outer layers of the skin, the hair, and the nails are composed of a tough, water-repellent protein called keratin.

Through its nerve endings, the skin serves as our principal organ of touch, and also allows us to perceive heat, cold, pain, and other stimuli. Sometimes, whether we like it or not, the skin reveals our innermost emotions, such as when we blush, turn pale, or become covered with goose bumps.

Skin also has important mechanical functions that affect other organs. For instance, the cholesterol in the skin absorbs sunlight to make vitamin D, which is needed for strong bones. The sebaceous glands deep within the skin manufacture and secrete lubricants to prevent evaporation of moisture and bodily fluids. The sweat glands moisten and cool the body with water and minerals secreted from the blood, thus acting as an important temperature-regulating mechanism.

SKIN AND THE OMEGA-3 FATTY ACIDS

Essential fatty acids are essential to your skin's health. Every cell in the skin—just as those in the rest of the body—is wrapped in a membrane, which consists mainly of substances derived from Omega-3 and Omega-6 fatty acids. The cell's efficiency and health depend largely on these membranes. When a serious essential fatty acid deficiency occurs, the flow of nutrients into and waste out of the cell is impeded. The manufacture of proteins and other cellular activities are also impeded because the cell can't work properly when the membranes are damaged.

Deficiencies in essential fatty acids have long been known to cause eczema—rough, bumpy scales and crusty, oozing skin—in children, and to make skin water-permeable, leading to excessive thirst. But my studies and the studies of other researchers show that such deficiencies can lead to a host of other skin problems as well.

Omega-3 fatty acids are particularly important in the skin functions of heat regulation, fat distribution, hair growth, and blood circulation. All of these functions are adaptations to life in a cold climate. As we saw in Chapter 2, plants make more Omega-3 fats, particularly ALA, in response to cold weather. This short-chain Omega-3 is converted by the body into the longer-chain Omega-3s that the skin needs to build healthy cell membranes. Therefore, people who live in a cold climate need more Omega-3s for healthy skin.

The Omega-3 fats are also needed to produce prostaglandins in the skin. Prostaglandins, the regulatory chemicals described in Chapter 2, are involved in the cellular activity that leads to both inflammation and healing. Groups of prostaglandins, formed from essential fatty acids, can trigger either process. When an Omega-3 deficiency occurs, too many of the prostaglandins that incite inflammation and too few of the ones that promote healing are available. The very rapid healing of the skin experienced by the volunteers in a study I conducted indicates that both the Omega-3 and the Omega-6 fatty acids are needed to maintain a balance in the skin's prostaglandins.

SKIN CHANGES IN THE FORTY-FOUR-PATIENT STUDY

I conducted a pilot study in the early 1980s to see if the Omega-3 oils could help ease a variety of ailments. The study itself, which involved forty-four patients, is described in Chapter 4. But some of the most dramatic results involved the easing of my volunteers' various skin problems.

On the basis of this study's results, I now think many skin ailments qualify as symptoms of an Omega-3 fatty acid deficiency, especially when seen in combination with other manifestations of the modern malnutrition described in Chapter 3. Chronic skin disorders, such as scaling, cracking, and persistent infections of the hair follicles, healed only after the volunteers began taking flaxseed oil, an oil high in Omega-3. The general color and elasticity of the volunteers' skin also improved greatly.

Skin Conditions Among the Volunteers

In addition to the other health complaints that prompted the patients to join the Omega-3 study, chronic skin problems plagued thirty-nine of the forty-four people involved, problems such as:

- Raw, cracked skin; chapped, raw knuckles and heels; and heavy callus formation

- Seborrheic dermatitis, a skin condition that is recognized by its flaking, red, patchy skin. It is evident in the formation of dandruff of the eyebrows, with patchy eczema around the eyes, nose, or cheeks, or on the outer ear canals

- Scaling of the skin on the scalp. Most subjects had non-stop dandruff that didn't respond fully to special shampoos or treatments

- Scaling of the skin on the shin and forearm, and flaking of the skin of the outer ear canal

- Sun sensitivity, including poor tanning with rapid sun-burning

- Alopecia areata, a sudden loss of hair in sharply defined patches, usually in the scalp or beard

- Phrynoderma—scaling and enlargement of the hair follicles—resulting in rough, prickly skin on the upper arms, elbows, thighs, and tips of the buttocks

- Acne

- Discoid lupus, thought to be an immune disorder related to standard lupus. It produces severe hair loss, scarring, and sun sensitivity

- Severe eczema of the hands

Many of the patients had suffered from these problems for years. Some had sought extensive medical treatment, but without any lasting relief.

The Response to Omega-3 Supplements

When the study volunteers were placed on the flaxseed-oil regimen, most noticed a rapid and marked smoothing and moisturizing of the hands—many saw positive results within a week.

As the healing continued, elbows, heels, and other parts of the body became smooth and soft. Within six weeks of the program's start, there was unmistakable improvement or even total disappearance of dandruff and flaky, dry skin on shins and forearms. Several subjects who were plagued in the winter by an unpleasant tingling of the skin following bathing or showering noticed that this reaction disappeared almost completely. Patchy red, flaking skin around the eyebrows, hairline, nose, and cheeks improved significantly.

Most exciting was the fact that skin texture, tone, and color improved—in one to four months—as did skin elasticity and firmness; even wrinkles were less pronounced. Sun sensitivity was lessened. A number of specific ailments also responded well.

Sudden Hair Loss Is Reversed

The patient with alopecia areata saw that condition improve. When coin-sized patches of hair suddenly fall out, alopecia areata is often the diagnosis. The onset of this frightening situation is often connected with great stress. Although in many individuals the hair loss may spontaneously reverse itself within a few months, many victims do not respond to conventional medical treatments, and the bald spots remain. This condition appears to benefit from modest doses of the antioxidant selenium, supplemental vitamins and minerals, and, above all, flaxseed oil over a period of six to twelve months.

My patient took these supplements for about a year. After four months, wispy, colorless "baby" hair appeared. After eight to nine months, the new hair began to take on adult pigmentation. After eighteen months, new hair was evident over all the patches.

Phrynoderma Roughness Made Smooth

Phrynoderma, also called follicular keratosis, looks like goose bumps, except that phrynoderma doesn't vanish when the shivering stops. To check whether you may have this very common skin condition, run your hands over your outer upper arms and elbows, thighs, and buttocks. The skin should be perfectly smooth. If you feel any roughness, you may have phrynoderma if the roughness is caused by hard, white flecks of dried skin within or on top of the hair follicles.

Nine of the ten volunteers in the study saw this condition clear up completely within a few months. Again, improvement appears to have resulted from reversing an Omega-3 deficiency. Within three weeks of starting on the flaxseed-oil supplements, the skin of the arms and thighs was smooth, and soon the skin on the buttocks grew smooth as well.

Acne Cleared Up

Acne results from an overproduction of skin oil by enlarged oil glands. This condition often occurs at puberty, when there is a sudden increase in hormone activity. If the enlarged and overactive oil glands become clogged, oil and other trapped secretions become home for bacteria. Blackheads and whiteheads form, and pimples become infected.

Today, physicians treat severe cases of acne with retinoic acid, a vitamin A derivative that has had remarkable effects in reducing acne. However, retinoic acid can only be used under a physician's care. It produces very unpleasant side effects, including severe skin damage, and has also been linked to birth defects.

In my study, three cases of acne in a single family improved solely with flaxseed oil. Other dramatic improvements were seen on a regimen of one to three capsules per day of a fish-oil supplement rich in Omega-3. All the patients affected by acne—aged twenty-two to thirty-six at the time of the study—had previously tried every accepted treatment, with only marginal benefits. The success of flaxseed oil, as well as that of retinoic acid, may be related to the fact that both vitamin A and the essential fatty acids are processed by the body in a similar manner.

Before trying the risky retinoic acid treatment for acne problems, I recommend four to six months on the low-risk Omega Program. Interestingly, some of the unpleasant effects of retinoic acid, such as drying of the lips, and elevation of cholesterol and fat levels in the blood, are problems that were corrected by Omega-3 supplementation. Some acne may respond best to a combination of the Omega-3 regimen and retinoic acid.

Discoid Lupus Symptoms Improved

Discoid lupus is not well understood by medical science. It is probably an immune disorder. The characteristic facial and upper body lesions resemble those found in the serious immune disorder systemic lupus erythematosus, but discoid lupus usually doesn't involve the whole body. Instead, it is generally confined to reddened, dried areas of damaged skin.

All discoid lupus treatment is largely experimental. One patient in my study, who had suffered from a severe case of discoid lupus for more than five years, had tried a number of treatments. He began to show improvement two weeks after starting the flaxseed-oil regimen, as his dry, leathery hands softened. By two months, his hands were reasonably normal, and the painful cracking had disappeared. For the first time, he could go out in the sun and actually tan normally. Most impressive was a growth of firmly rooted hair on the 40 percent of the scalp that had not been irreversibly scarred.

That the flaxseed oil caused the improvements was very clear. When the patient stopped taking the oil for only two weeks, his skin began to dry and his facial lesions returned.

The situation improved again when he resumed the oil supplements.

Eczema Significantly Reduced

Eczema is a general term that refers to itching and inflamed, scaling, oozing skin. It is a synonym for dermatitis, which means "inflammation of the skin." No one knows why some people suffer this hard-to-treat condition, which may be allergic and is often accompanied by hay fever or asthma. In rare cases, it can last a lifetime. About 7 million people in the United States are afflicted with eczema.

Eczema was significantly relieved in more than half of the study volunteers who had it.

OMEGA NUTRITION FOR YOUR SKIN'S HEALTH

The skin problems that result from a diet deficient in essential fatty acids—such as eczema, scaling, plugged hair follicles, and hair loss—are similar to those seen when certain B vitamins are missing in the diet. For example, pellagra—as we saw in Chapter 1—arises from a deficiency of niacin, a B vitamin. And pellagra is also associated with eczema and dry skin problems.

What do the B vitamins and essential fatty acids have in common that makes a deficiency of either—or both—produce skin problems? One of the fundamental functions of the B vitamins is to help convert shorter-chain fatty acids into longer-chain ones (see Chapter 2). The B vitamins then help to convert those longer fatty acids into prostaglandins. When either the B vitamins or the essential fatty acids are deficient, various kinds of skin problems occur.

Scientists have learned that zinc is another substance important for skin health, as a result of research into a childhood disease called acrodermatitis enteropathica. Infants born with this disease failed to grow normally and usually died in infancy. They suffered from an eczemalike skin rash, hair loss, and diarrhea. Researchers found that the disease is caused by an inability to absorb the essential trace mineral zinc. Fortunately, a simple cure was found. Treating such infants with supplemental zinc resulted in complete remission of the disease.

Researchers have noticed that hair loss and skin defects—such as abnormal skin permeability (leaky skin), inadequate healing of wounds, and immune disorders—can arise from a shortage of either essential fatty acids or zinc in the diet. The connection between zinc and Omega-3 resembles the connection between the B-vitamin complex and Omega-3. Like the B vitamins, zinc works in conjunction with cell enzymes that convert the short-chain essential fatty acids into longer-chain fats, some of which become prostaglandins.

Many of the ailments induced by this deficiency respond best when both zinc *and* essential fatty acids are introduced into the diet, either in foods or via supplements. This is another example of the powerful effects shown by essential nutrients working together.

Omega-3 also helps to keep skin healthy by helping cholesterol do its job. Cholesterol attaches itself to essential fatty acids, and thus becomes a stabilizing element of cell membranes in the skin and throughout the body. In an Omega-oil deficiency, cholesterol is forced to link up with saturated fats instead of essential fatty acids. The stabilizing effect disappears and weak, leaky cell membranes result. This defect creates abnormal permeability in the skin, which allows cell moisture to evaporate.

AN OMEGA SKIN-IMPROVEMENT PROGRAM

The Omega Program produced striking improvements in

the skin of most volunteers in the forty-four-patient study, and is described in detail in Chapters 11 and 12. Although good results were obtained initially on flaxseed oil alone, long-term improvement was reinforced by adding the nutrients described in those chapters. These nutrients include vitamin A (and vitamin A's precursor, beta-carotene), the B vitamins, and trace minerals such as selenium. These nutrients are what I call the Omega-3 cofactors, because the body requires them in order to properly use the Omega-3 fatty acids.

The skin improvements that can result from following the Omega Program include softer, smoother, firmer, seamless skin and thicker, fuller hair. The program can't make time stand still, but it can allow your body to deal with the changes that time brings. In short, the Omega Program provides a program of nutritional cosmetology— from the inside out.

CHAPTER 7

OMEGA NUTRITION AND REPRODUCTIVE HEALTH

M ore than in other areas of health, reproductive health reflects a complex interplay of hormones and organs, an interplay affected by diet. Problems such as premenstrual syndrome and infertility can reflect deficiencies in the essential fatty acids. These deficiencies can be corrected through the use of Omega-3 supplements. In this chapter, we will see how diet affects the sexual health of both women and men, and why good nutrition is important for prospective parents.

FEMALE SEXUAL HEALTH AND OMEGA-3

The functions of a woman's reproductive system—menstruation, pregnancy, menopause—often place demands on her body that require extra nutritional support. Also, many nutritional imbalances are related to ailments common in women, such as anemia, breast cancer, osteoporosis, migraine headache, and premenstrual syndrome. And, of course, a woman's health during pregnancy determines the health of her child.

The Omega-3 oils form an important component of a woman's sexual health. In the forty-four-patient Omega-3 study I conducted in the early 1980s (see Chapter 4), three women who had suffered menstrual irregularity for many years started having regular periods after a number of months on supplements of flaxseed oil, a rich Omega-3 source. In addition, many of these women's other health problems, such as arthritis and bursitis, improved when they took the flaxseed-oil supplements.

Let's see how the Omega-3 fatty acids can help ease premenstrual syndrome, menstrual cramps, infertility, and menopausal problems. For more information on the Omega Program, see Chapters 11 and 12.

Premenstrual Syndrome

Many women experience occasional discomfort before their periods start. But women with premenstrual syndrome (PMS) experience a pattern of various discomforts, some of which can be quite severe. It is most likely to be severe in women who have undergone a change in their levels of estrogen and progesterone, the primary female hormones, or who are between the ages of thirty and forty-five. Many women who have PMS also have irregular menstrual cycles.

PMS includes some or all of the following symptoms:

- Nervous tension, mood swings, anxiety, crying, and anger

- Breast pain or tenderness

- Fatigue, dizziness, forgetfulness, headache

- Inability to sleep soundly

- Food cravings, especially for sweet or salty foods

The exact cause of PMS is unknown. It could be triggered by any or all of certain imbalances:

- In hormone levels—too much estrogen and too little progesterone

- In levels of different prostaglandins—the regulatory chemicals described in Chapter 2

- In brain chemicals called neurotransmitters that pass messages from one nerve cell to another

All of these factors are closely linked.

Physicians once dismissed PMS as a emotional reaction to a nonexistent problem. But we now know that PMS is real, and is treatable. Omega-3 fatty acids play an important part in rebalancing the prostaglandins. The Omega-3s discourage the production of prostaglandins that irritate nerves and tissues while encouraging the production of prostaglandins that soothe the body. Prostaglandins translate the messages of hormones, including estrogen and progesterone, into a format that cells can use. Prostaglandins also coordinate the operations of the nervous system, including those of the neural circuits in the brain. Flaxseed and fish oils provide the essential fatty acids needed to keep the prostaglandin system in balance, which in turn reduces or eliminates PMS symptoms.

Menstrual Cramps

Almost all women experience some cramping in the lower abdomen during their periods. But some women suffer cramps, often accompanied by lower back pain and leg aches, severe enough to make them miserable for several days each month.

These cramps are caused by contractions of the uterus. The uterus contracts in response to prostaglandins produced by the Omega-6 fatty acids. If there is too much Omega-6 in the diet, and not enough Omega-3—a common occurrence in the modern diet—the contractions can become excessive. Drugs that interfere with the production of Omega-6 prostaglandins also, unfortunately, hinder production of prostaglandins that relax the muscles. Taking Omega-3 supplements for one week before, and during, each menstrual period can allow the body to make less of the prostaglandins that cause contraction, and more of the ones that cause relaxation.

Infertility

One cause of female infertility is a thickening of the cervical mucus, which impedes the movement of sperm. Another is that some vaginal secretions act as spermicides. In both cases, a deficiency in essential fatty acids may contribute to the problem.

In animal studies, adding both Omega-3 and Omega-6 fats to the diet produced an increase in fertility greater than could be achieved through use of either supplement by itself. The Omega oils work together to make secretions thinner and more fluid, and to ensure that the secretions provide a hospitable environment for sperm.

In my Omega-3 study, one woman—who had borne twins four years earlier only after taking fertility drugs—had not had a normal period for ten years. She also suffered from a number of other health problems, including dry skin and arthritis. Two weeks after she started taking flaxseed oil to relieve her arthritis, she had some surprising results: she started menstruating normally again. Seven months later, to her delight, she became pregnant without the use of hormonal drugs of any kind. While taking an average of one tablespoon of flaxseed oil and the usual Omega Program-recommended supplements every day, she had an uneventful pregnancy and delivered a healthy baby boy. This was our first flaxseed-oil baby, from preconception through breastfeeding (a topic that is covered in Chapter 8).

Vaginal Dryness Associated With Menopause

After menopause, dwindling female hormones cause diminished vaginal lubrication and a general thinning of vaginal tissues. This problem bothers many women. In addition to the dryness itself, the symptoms may include itching, irritation, urinary incontinence, and pain during intercourse.

These symptoms are usually treated with hormone replacement therapy. But for many women, these synthetic hormones produce unpleasant and sometimes serious side effects, including gallbladder disease, persistent headache, blood clots in the brain or lungs, and a higher risk for breast cancer.

Inadequate vaginal lubrication may be avoidable, to a large extent, when the body's Omega-oil balance is right. All bodily secretions depend on how well each secretory cell functions. Essential fatty acids provide the molecules needed to build healthy secretory cells, including those in the glands that lubricate and moisten vaginal tissues. Two of the women in my study reported an increase in vaginal secretions after a few months of flaxseed-oil supplements.

MALE SEXUAL HEALTH AND OMEGA-3

Many researchers have observed that male fertility, as reflected in sperm counts, has declined precipitously in just a few decades—there's been close to a 50 percent dropoff. One possible factor in this decline is exposure to numerous industrial and agricultural chemicals that behave like estrogen within men's bodies. For example, the insecticide DDT, which has persisted in the environment despite having been banned in 1972, mimics female sex hormones and could have a feminizing effect on male fetuses. They may then grow into adult men with lower sperm counts and other sexual anomalies. The introduction of DDT in the 1940s coincided with today's increasing reports of male reproductive problems. Furthermore, DDT breaks down in the body into a chemical that inhibits androgens, the male sex hormones.

A major cause of reproductive disorders in animals is known to be an essential fatty acid deficiency. Is it possible the same is true for humans?

A dietary deficiency of Omega-6 essential fatty acids was rare among the men (and women) in my forty-four-patient study, but an Omega-3 deficiency was common. For healthy sexual and reproductive function, the testes, or male sex glands, normally contain a great concentration of the long-chain Omega-3 called DHA. The body can make DHA out of other short-chain Omega-3s (see Chapter 2), or it can get ready-made DHA from the diet, mainly from seafood.

Several of the men in my study reported an increase in sex drive while on the Omega Program. This supports the folklore belief that oysters are a virility food, since oysters and all shellfish contain DHA and another Omega-3 oil, EPA. Oysters are also a rich source of zinc, a mineral vital to a man's reproductive health.

Omega-3 fatty acids may also provide a solution for another health problem common to men called benign prostatic hypertrophy, or enlarged prostate gland. The condition interferes with sleep because the prostate often swells to the point where it presses on the urethra, with the result that the patient awakes several times a night to urinate. The condition can also interfere with sexual potency.

Today, enlarged prostate is so common in men over forty that it is considered an unavoidable, irreversible symptom of middle age. But is this natural, or is this just another disorder caused by distortions in the modern diet?

Two men in my Omega-3 study who had suffered for about a year from this prostate problem recovered completely on the flaxseed-oil program. A third man was a physician who published an article in a medical journal about his experience—he felt that flaxseed oil actually saved him from imminent prostate surgery.

For information on the Omega Program, see Chapters 11 and 12.

PREGNANCY, NUTRITION, AND OMEGA-3

Both mothers *and* fathers need good nutrition to ensure healthy babies. If both are on a healthy diet before conception, one full of natural, unprocessed foods, no other dietary controls are necessary.

However, most people live on what I call the Great American Experimental Diet of too much refined flour and sugar, and not enough vitamins, minerals, and other essential nutrients. The effects of alcohol, drugs, nicotine, caffeine, and stress during pregnancy have been widely studied. Clearly, it is best for the mother and the father to avoid all these things. However, there has not been enough emphasis on preconception nutrition, especially on the nutritional missing link—the Omega-3 fatty acids.

In this section, I will first explain why the essential fatty acids are so important to the developing fetus. Then, I will discuss the role of natural foods—including Omega-oil supplements—in diets for pregnant mothers. Finally, I'll give you a list of dietary steps you can take to give yourself the best possible chance of having a healthy baby. For information on the Omega Program, see Chapters 11 and 12.

Nutrition and Prenatal Development

The essential fatty acids play important roles in helping the fetus to develop properly. One role is in the development of the immune system, which is programed during fetal life and in the early months after birth. As we've seen in previous chapters, the essential fatty acids are important to the immune system's functioning. If a pregnant woman eats a diet that overlooks the Omega-3 fatty acids, as commonly happens today, the developing child can suffer illnesses—both mental and physical—related to a weakened immune system, along with other problems.

Essential fatty acids may play their most important role, though, in the development of the fetal brain. In 1968, Swedish scientist Lars Svennerholm showed that DHA, an important Omega-3 fat, was the major unsaturated fat in the brain, and that the Omega-6 fat ARA was second in prominence. (For information on the different types of fats, see Chapter 2.) Scientists realized that the fetal brain depended on fatty acids that had to come from the mother, either through her diet or from her own tissues. The fetus, while it could make certain fats, could not create these essential fatty acids by itself.

As early as 1971, Italian scientist C. Galli and his colleagues emphasized the importance of supplying both Omega-6 and Omega-3 fatty acids in the diets of pregnant women. They said a malnourished fetus who was denied these fats could suffer "significant, perhaps irreversible developmental damage to the brain." These findings have been verified by other studies.

Why Fish and Fish Oil May Be Brain Food

During the last trimester of pregnancy, the fetus's brain undergoes a tremendous growth spurt, for which large amounts of Omega-3 DHA and Omega-6 ARA are needed. When a vegetarian mother-to-be consumes nuts, seeds, grains and oils that supply linoleic acid, the first member of the Omega-6 family, her body's enzymes are able to convert linoleic acid into enough ARA to take care of both her needs and the needs of her baby.

However, even if a pregnant vegetarian consumes foods rich in ALA, the first member of the Omega-3 family, her body may not be able to convert ALA into enough DHA to cover both her own needs, which are greater during pregnancy, and those of her baby. DHA is present in seafood, but if the woman cannot or will not eat seafood, she can get the DHA she and her baby need from fish oil, or from newer products that derive DHA from algae (see "DHA From Sea Vegetables" on page 61).

By the way, DHA is not only needed in large amounts by the developing brain, but also by the eyes, and, if the baby is a boy, by the testes. Maybe that's why the practice of giving cod-liver oil to pregnant women has such a long tradition. For a possible explanation as to why seafood is such an important source of nutrients in humans, see "Are We Genetically Designed for High Omega-3 Intake?" on page 90.

Eating to Make Healthy Babies

Like everyone else, pregnant women are adversely affected by the deficiencies of the modern, industrialized diet. Much of our knowledge in this field comes from the early work of Weston A. Price, a dentist and anthropologist

Are We Genetically Designed for High Omega-3 Intake?

Human beings require more than twice as much energy, in proportion to our body size, to fuel our brains as does any other species. We now know that normal fetal brain development relies heavily on the availability of two essential fatty acids, ARA and DHA, that are not found in many land-based food sources. However, DHA exists abundantly in aquatic plants and animals, and ARA is found in shellfish.

British scientist Sir Alister Hardy broke with accepted evolutionary theory in 1961, when he speculated that early humans may have descended from apes that left the trees, not for the African grasslands—as most scientists suggest—but for the shores of lakes and seas! He thought that these "aquatic apes" learned to walk by wading in the water, and to use tools by using rocks to crack open shells. Eventually, over millions of years, early humans developed characteristics not found in other primates, or in most land animals. For example, humans have little body hair, a special diving reflex, and a layer of fat underneath the skin. These are all typical features of sea mammals, such as dolphins and seals.

Humans also have large brains in proportion to the size of their bodies—a large brain-to-body ratio. Most large mammals have low brain-to-body ratios. For instance, the ox and the elephant share a brain-to-body ratio one-twentieth of ours; the gorilla, one-sixth of ours. The only large mammals that have kept a high brain-to-body ratio are those living in the sea. British scientist Michael Crawford has suggested that the brain of the aquatic ape was able to keep pace as body size increased because there was an abundance of high-energy aquatic foods that contained the fatty acids the brain required. Neither the grasslands nor the forest offered that much in the way of brain-building foodstuffs.

who examined the diet and health of people in preindustrial cultures. From the late 1920s through the 1930s, Price and his wife, Florence, analyzed food samples, did dental examinations, and took at least 18,000 photographs of people living in traditional cultures in places such as Alaska, Peru, Australia, and Africa.

The Prices were impressed by the general health, including the superb dental health, of these peoples, and by how all of these societies took special pains to ensure that pregnant and breastfeeding women received ample nourishment. In many of these cultures, pregnant women ate fish, shellfish, and aquatic plants. In all of them, the diet offered a wide variety of both plant and animal foods that we now understand to be good sources of Omega-3 and Omega-6 fats. Often, tribes would travel great distances or even exchange food with enemies to obtain a varied diet.

However, when the Prices revisited these cultures years later, after these peoples had abandoned traditional diets for white flour and sugary foods, they found rampant disease and tooth decay. The evidence showed that when the diets of these preindustrial peoples were modernized, so were their diseases.

Watching your diet can help you improve your chances of giving birth to a healthy, happy baby. (For a word of caution about special diets, see page 92). Follow these guidelines—after discussing them with your physician— when planning a pregnancy:

- For at least six months before conception, both the woman and the man should choose foods that supply an abundance of Omega-3 and Omega-6 fatty acids, in the form of foods from temperate and cold climates. This includes fish, such as salmon and bluefish; nuts, such as walnuts; grains, such as winter wheat; and oils, such as flaxseed.

A Word of Caution to Mothers on Special Diets

From conception to birth, a prospective mother who is suffering from a health disorder should be treated with dietary supplements as well as with appropriate medication. But what kind of and how much supplementation is a complex problem, since the supplement program that is best for the mother's health may not be best for the fetus. Probably the best compromise in such cases is to decrease the mother's supplement program to the lowest possible level that still provides minimum control over her illness. Problems this complex must be worked out in consultation with a physician and a nutritionist.

- Before and after conception, the woman should consume a diet high in not only essential fatty acids, but in fiber, vitamins, and minerals as well. Multivitamin and multimineral supplements that include folic acid, selenium, manganese, calcium, zinc, and chromium are important.

- Most women should gain close to three pounds a month, or between twenty-five to thirty-five pounds over nine months. A woman should *never* attempt to lose weight during pregnancy.

- During pregnancy, the woman should increase the number of calories she eats to about 10 to 15 percent above her normal level. For example, if she usually consumes about 2,200 calories, an increase of about 300 calories—for a total of 2,500 calories—should be her new daily intake. She should get her additional calories mainly from fish and chicken.

REPRODUCTIVE HEALTH AND OMEGA-3

Both women and men need adequate amounts of Omega-3 oil for good reproductive health. In women, Omega-3 can help regulate periods and ease the discomfort of menopause. In men, it can help relieve the swelling of the prostate that so many men seem to think of as a natural consequence of growing older. In both sexes, it can help some forms of infertility.

If you are a parent-to-be—or planning to become one—why not give your baby the best possible start? Proper nutrition is important for your child to grow and develop normally, and getting adequate amounts of the Omega-3 fatty acids is an important part of proper nutrition. I urge you to discuss these issues with your physician.

CHAPTER 8

THE OMEGA-STRONG INFANT AND TODDLER

A s an adult, you have to cope with the body you've got—and deal with any weaknesses you may have developed as a result of an Omega-deficient diet in your formative years. But the mistakes of the past need not be repeated. By recognizing your child's complete nutritional needs, you can give your offspring a bright start. In this chapter, we'll first look at several childhood problems that may be linked to an Omega-oil deficiency. I'll then tell you how you can use Omega oils to help keep your infant or toddler healthy.

OMEGA DEFICIENCY IN EARLY CHILDHOOD

The effects of a deficiency in essential fatty acids in pregnancy and infancy can make themselves obvious early. For example, extended colic in infants can be a juvenile form of the adult irritable bowel syndrome.

Many disorders of the digestive system originate from an imbalance in the Omega-3 and Omega-6 fatty acids, which results in an imbalance in the regulatory chemicals, called prostaglandins, that these fatty acids produce (see Chapter 2). In particular, certain Omega-6 prostaglandins can create irritation or inflammation, unless kept in check by Omega-3 fats. Since all cells and tissues can produce prostaglandins, the inflammatory kind may target not only a child's digestive system, but also the skin, the bronchial passages, or even the brain.

Sudden Infant Death Syndrome

Sudden infant death syndrome (SIDS), commonly called crib death, has always been a puzzling syndrome. The name describes what happens with no hint as to why—infants die without warning from unknown causes.

In a very high number of SIDS cases, the infants were lying on their stomachs, which may interfere with swallowing and breathing. SIDS appears to have some of the same features as a disorder involving the swallowing reflex suffered by several adults in my forty-four-patient study (see Chapter 4). The adults, who were deficient in Omega-3, would suddenly be unable to breathe, often to the point of almost suffocating.

Studies of crib death show that:

- A high number of SIDS infants were on formulas that lacked Omega-3 fatty acids.

- Formulas often contain very low levels of biotin, a vitamin the body needs to process fatty acids. Cow's milk is low in biotin.

- Several autopsies showed low blood levels of vitamin E

and selenium, which are needed to protect the essential fatty acids from rancidity.

Low levels of Omega-3 fats, biotin, and selenium in infant formulas result in infants who are malnourished. Malnutrition doesn't always cause obvious problems, such as slow growth or poor weight gain. It can be far more insidious, subtly affecting all aspects of health and behavior. Therefore, I an convinced that malnutrition may put an infant at risk for SIDS. Recent autopsy studies have pinpointed the presence of abnormal brain chemistry in SIDS victims. One wonders: could adequate Omega-3 intake by the mother help to prevent brain abnormalities before the baby is born?

Attention-Deficit Hyperactivity Disorder

Attention-deficit hyperactivity disorder (ADHD) is the term used to describe children who are chronically inattentive, impulsive, and hyperactive—to such a degree that they create real problems at home and in school. As ADHD children grow up, they are more likely than other children to drop out of high school or develop antisocial behavior.

ADHD children also tend to have more allergies, eczema, asthma, headaches, stomachaches, ear infections, and dry skin than non-ADHD youngsters. These problems are among the problems related to modernization-disease syndrome—the syndrome that arises from malnutrition centered on an Omega-3 deficiency (see Chapter 3). The connection between Omega-3 and ADHD has been confirmed by studies in which youngsters with ADHD, when compared with non-ADHD children, had much lower blood levels of DHA, an Omega-3 fat. DHA is necessary for normal function of both the eye and the brain's cerebral cortex, the part of the brain that handles higher functions such as reasoning and memory. Also, ADHD affects many more boys than girls, and boys require more Omega-3 both before and after birth.

The number of ADHD children in the United States keeps going up. Is it a coincidence that this rise has occurred at the same time as a huge rise in the trans-fatty acid content of packaged foods and fast foods? As you will recall from Chapters 2 and 3, trans-fatty acids are produced when oil is hydrogenated. These "funny fats" displace essential fatty acids within the body, making it more difficult for the essential fats to do their jobs. Unfortunately, bakery goods, French fries, chips, and other snacks that children love are full of trans-fatty acids. For vulnerable ADHD children, trans-fatty acids may even cause lower blood levels of DHA and other essential fats.

Children with ADHD may have trouble converting the short-chain essential fatty acids into longer-chain Omega-3 and Omega-6 fats (see Chapter 2). Therefore, these youngsters benefit from getting ready-made DHA, a long-chain fat, in the form of fatty fish or fish oil. Evening primrose oil provides the Omega-6 fat GLA, which may bypass a blocked Omega-6 conversion step. Together, they offer a healthier balance of Omega-3 and Omega-6 in brain and body tissues, and a lessened output of the "bad" prostaglandins that foster discomfort and irritability. (For information on the use of these oils, see Chapters 11 and 12.)

Autism and the Immune System

Autism is a mysterious and heartbreaking ailment. Autistic babies don't respond normally to being cuddled and cared for. As toddlers and young children, they tend to live in a world of their own, seemingly indifferent to people but morbidly attached to objects. Comfortable only when endlessly repeating rituals, they usually appear to be overwhelmed by the noise and activity of normal childhood play. Many autistic children never develop speech; others use language oddly, repeating phrases over and over, or are unable to link thoughts through language.

In 1985, scientists at Stanford University discovered evidence that connected autism with an immune system abnormality. Researchers noted the presence of an unusual antibody—a substance usually produced by the immune system in response to an infection—circulating in the blood and spinal fluid of autistic children. This antibody may interfere with brain chemistry by interrupting messages normally communicated by a substance called serotonin.

Could the rise of autism be related to modern malnutrition, especially to a prevalent Omega-3 deficiency? The immune system requires both Omega-3 and Omega-6 fats, but the modern diet contains much more Omega-6 than Omega-3. Studies show that autistic children improve when given supplements of vitamin B6 and magnesium, both of which are needed if essential fatty acids are to be used properly within the body. I an convinced that adding Omega-3 fatty acids to the diet can help both brain function and the immune system, and thus help fight autism.

Dental Problems

Crooked, crowded teeth and an overbite—the upper teeth coming down too far over the lowers—are seen in the first teeth of tiny toddlers as well as in those of older children. Suggested causes range from heredity to chronic thumb-sucking or mouth-breathing.

In the 1920s and 1930s, noted researcher and dentist Dr. Weston A. Price (see Chapter 7) and his wife investigated the connection between diet and dental health in preindustrial societies. Traveling to remote areas, they examined native people for signs of dental and other health problems. They described the people they encountered as generally vigorous, healthy, and free of dental problems. The native diets were good sources of fiber and other essential nutrients, including ample amounts of the Omega-3 fats. To the Prices, the nutrition connection was unmistakable.

But when they visited the same groups years later, rampant tooth decay—along with other diseases of modern society—had appeared wherever people had given up traditional diets in favor of modern foods such as refined sugar and flour. And the children of mothers who had abandoned the traditional diet had narrowed faces and jaws, pinched nostrils, overbite, and crooked, crowded teeth.

Could the foods we eat affect our jaws and teeth in just a few short generations? Medical opinions vary, but we do know that fiber, vitamins, minerals, and Omega-3 fatty acids were more abundant in human diets thousands of years ago, as they were in the earlier diets of the people the Prices studied. This may explain why skulls of ancient people typically have generous facial bones with sound, well-spaced teeth.

BREASTFEEDING AND THE OMEGA PROGRAM

Unless there is the most compelling reason for not breastfeeding, mothers should breastfeed their infants for at least six months after birth, and preferably for up to two years. There is no comparable substitute. A well-nourished nursing mother provides her infant with a perfect blend of fatty acids for fast-growing brain and body tissues. A mother's milk also supplies important antibodies and antimicrobial factors that guard her baby against disease and infection. Neither cow's milk nor infant formula offers this protection. This assumes, of course, that the mother is eating a diet rich in the nutrients that are often missing from the modern diet (see Chapter 3).

The premature infant especially needs breast milk for its immature system. I know several mothers of "preemies" who, unable to nurse, hired wet nurses or secured human milk for their babies. The results were well worth the trouble. Breast milk not only supplies antibodies to protect the tiny preemie, but also provides the long-chain Omega-3 and Omega-6 fats needed for growth.

In this section, we'll first see how good nutrition for you can translate into good nutrition for your baby. And if you can't breastfeed, we'll see how you can boost the nutritional value of the formula you use.

Good Nutrition for Mother Means Good Nutrition for Baby

Infants need fats in different amounts and for different purposes than adults do. For example, we adults can manage well with little or no cholesterol in our diet because the body makes enough of it to take care of all our needs. An infant, on the other hand, requires quite a lot of cholesterol but may not yet be able to make enough. In its rapidly growing brain, for instance, cholesterol forms 30 percent of the brain's structure, which is largely fat-based. Infants need cholesterol not just for brain growth, but to also strengthen all cell membranes, waterproof the skin, make vitamin D from sunlight, make bile acids, and so on.

For this reason, mother's milk is high in cholesterol. In fact, infants and toddlers do not benefit from a low-cholesterol diet, regardless of its purported benefits for older children and adults.

The brain does a lot of growing before and after birth. A fetus is mostly head and brain—the brain uses 70 percent of the fetus's energy! Yet skull size is limited by the size of the birth canal. So, in order for the brain to reach its full capacity, it continues to grow for many months after birth.

The brain consumes 60 percent of the infant's energy intake, compared with 20 percent of an adult's. While the brains of other primates double in weight after birth, the human baby quadruples its brain weight by about the age of eighteen months.

This brain growth requires, in addition to cholesterol, sufficient amounts of the polyunsaturated Omega fatty acids. Milk from well-nourished mothers provides the infant with the Omega fats DHA and ARA, in the correct proportions, along with other required nutrients. As we saw in Chapter 7, DHA and ARA are the principal building blocks of the brain and of other tissues throughout the body.

These Omega fats are especially important for premature, or preterm, babies—those born before the full nine-month term. In Chapter 7, we saw that the fetus cannot convert the short-chain essential fatty acids into the long-chain ones, DHA and ARA, that are needed to build brain tissue. This means that preemies do not yet have the ability to make enough DHA and ARA to make up for the rich supply they would have gotten within the womb. Even full-term babies may not be able to do this conversion efficiently. Thus, the value of providing young infants with the benefits of breast milk is becoming increasingly clear to medical researchers.

Mother's milk can have drawbacks if the mother's diet is lacking in nutrients such as the Omega-3 fats, the minerals selenium and zinc, and the vitamin biotin. The absence of certain nutrients in breast milk indicates a lack of those nutrients in the mother's diet. Sadly, the breast milk of many mothers in the United States reflects the poor nutrient value of the average American diet. American mothers produce milk that often has only one-fourth of the Omega-3 DHA found in milk from mothers who eat traditional diets.

If you plan to nurse your baby, you must eat a diet rich in the nutrients your child needs. First, remember that you need more calories, anywhere from 500 to 1,000 more calories each day than you ate before you became pregnant. For example, if your usual intake had been 2,200 calories, you would need to increase it to between 2,700 and 3,200 calories a day while nursing. (If you're worried about gaining weight, see "Weight Loss—Another Breast-feeding Plus" on page 104.)

I would also encourage you to take supplements that contain adequate amounts of the essential fatty acids, especially the Omega-3 fats that the modern diet generally lacks. One or more tablespoons of flaxseed oil, plus one teaspoon of cod-liver oil or several fish-oil capsules, will ensure that your milk has a plentiful supply of the essential fatty acids. If you're looking for a complete supplement program, see Chapters 11 and 12 for a description of the Omega Program.

If You Can't Breastfeed—Omega-Fortified Formula

Everyone, including formula makers, agrees that the ideal formula is one that achieves a nutrient and fatty-acid balance close to that of mother's milk. Three critical long-chain fatty acids in breast milk are Omega-3 DHA and Omega-6 ARA and GLA. While these fats are added to formulas made in other countries, they are not being added to formulas made in this country, although American manufacturers are considering the addition of DHA and ARA to preemie formula. Maybe letters or phone calls from mothers to formula makers in the United States, asking that they follow the lead of firms in places such as Japan and Korea, might speed up the process!

Manufacturers debate the need for the addition of such fats. But that's not surprising, because up to 1990, these

Weight Loss— Another Breastfeeding Plus

Breastfeeding is not only good for your baby's health, it's good for your shape. A nursing mother requires about 10 to 15 percent more calories and nutrients than she did during pregnancy. Not only does nursing burn up calories, it also stimulates uterine contraction, which in turn encourages the uterus to return to its normal size. This allows the nursing mother to return to her prepregnancy weight and shape more rapidly than a mother who formula-feeds her infant.

companies' scientists also questioned the need for the primary Omega-3 fat, ALA. As a matter of fact, up until the late 1960s, many infants in the United States developed severe eczema because formulas lacked not only ALA but also the primary Omega-6 fat, linoleic acid. Now, at least, most formulas include both.

Until long-chain fatty acids are added to infant formula, mothers who are unable to breastfeed may have to add DHA to each day's formula supply in the form of five to ten drops of cod-liver oil. It's not ideal—cod-liver oil has no GLA and very little ARA—but it has been used safely for years. Another option may be an algae-based vegetarian source of DHA (see page 61). In addition, you could improve your baby's formula by squeezing one or two capsules of evening primrose oil into the day's supply (one capsule supplies about 40 milligrams of GLA). You can also watch for new formulas that contain a better balance of the Omega fatty acids—see "Vegetarian Fatty-Acid Supplements Available" on page 106.

Human milk is best for babies. It is always preferable, even to any new, improved formulas. It is rewarding, however, to observe that pressure from conscientious scientists in Europe, the United States, and Asia is spurring the development of a sensible, safe way to improve the fatty-acid content of formula.

THE OMEGA TODDLER DIET

Good nutrition continues to be important as your child moves from the infant to the toddler stage. Start your baby on the right foods by encouraging a taste for high-Omega and high-fiber foods.

Solid foods should be started no earlier than six months of age, to avoid either crowding out milk or provoking sensitivities to foods that a baby's immature digestive system is not yet ready to handle. When your baby starts on solid food, use only foods that are low in sugar, hydrogenated oils, and southern-grown oils. (For information on the different types of oils, see Chapter 2.) Omega oils—cod-liver, soy, wheat germ, walnut, or flaxseed—are the preferred sources of essential fatty acids in your baby's diet.

Between six and ten months, you may gradually introduce solids. To be on the safe side, especially if there are allergies in the family, offer the baby only one bite or one-half teaspoon of a new food the first day, slowly increasing the amount during the next few days. Don't introduce more than one new food over a five-day period. This way, you can make sure that each new item is well tolerated. Avoid cereals, as babies do not digest starches well at this age.

When your baby is nine to ten months of age, you can add cooked egg yolk, then gradually introduce cooked egg white. Usually, cottage cheese is accepted, and at this time you can add small pieces of fish, fowl, or lamb—lamb liver is an especially good source of iron. At one year, the baby should be getting about a quart of breast milk or formula

Vegetarian Fatty-Acid Supplements Available

Purified vegetarian sources of the Omega fats DHA and ARA are now available to the makers of infant formula. Martek Biosciences Corporation of Columbia, Maryland has granted licenses to approximately 40 percent of the world's producers of infant formula, allowing them to incorporate these fatty acids into their products. Manufacturers in Belgium were the first to use the vegetarian DHA and ARA in formulas designed just for preterm infants.

daily, plus at least three meals and several snacks. Other good starter foods are oatmeal, applesauce and other cooked fruits, and mashed, steamed vegetables such as carrots, beets, yams, and squash. Basically, you will be feeding your child from your own table.

Baby food should be prepared without sugar and salt. The infant's natural taste for sweets is well satisfied by the sugar that is in milk and by naturally sweet fruits and vegetables. Mothers can save their children from a losing battle with sugar cravings later on by understanding this, and by sticking firmly to the principle of no sweets. Added salt is not required either, since milk and other foods provide plenty of salt to meet the baby's needs.

The one-year-old can eat a variety of foods from the family's standard Omega-3 diet as long as the food is mashed or cut into small pieces. Cod-liver or other fish oil—five to ten drops by dropper or teaspoon—should be given.

Fresh orange juice and puréed fruits are usually a welcome addition to the one-year-old's diet. You can dissolve vitamin C powder into juice or puréed fruits without a noticeable flavor change whenever you want to give your baby extra vitamin C. Breast milk and formula contain small amounts of vitamin C, so many parents are choosing to use supplements of 50 to 100 milligrams a day.

By the time the baby has four molars—generally at twelve to eighteen months of age—and can chew reasonably well, steamed vegetables should be served fork-tender instead of mushy, and raw fruits can be added to the diet. Peanuts and other nuts are too easy to choke on at this age, but Omega nut butters are a valuable food for the baby.

By the time the child is three and has all twenty baby teeth, raw vegetables and fresh unsalted nuts and seeds—for example, walnuts, almonds, chestnuts, hazel nuts, sunflower seeds, and pumpkin seeds—can be a readily accepted part of the day's meals and snacks. At this age, your child will most likely be eating most of the foods in the family's diet.

Ample fiber intake is important for bowel training because sufficient dietary fiber prevents constipation. As the baby gradually eats more fiber in the form of vegetables, whole-grain cereals, beans, and fruit, constipation should not be a problem. If it is, a teaspoon of unprocessed bran or one-third teaspoon of flaxseed meal—given with puréed fruit or yogurt, or added to cereals—should allow formation of well-shaped bowel movements that are passed effortlessly.

STARTING OMEGA HEALTH EARLY

All the evidence points to breast milk as the primary and best source of nutrition for babies, since it provides the essential fatty acids that are critical for good health, both in childhood and throughout life. Since the 1980s, a great rush of worldwide interest in the Omega-3 fats has produced more than 5,000 studies. Many of them explore the ways in which Omega-3 affects nerve and brain development in infant animals. For instance, we've learned that Omega-3 DHA in the eye's retina is needed to convert incoming images into swift electrical signals to the brain. It's not surprising, then, that a deficiency of DHA in the diet of infant monkeys causes them to lose keenness in their vision, and to have slower responses to visual signals. Although studies with human infants are difficult, and therefore scarce, they show that preterm babies on either breast milk or DHA-fortified formula could process visual images faster than babies on DHA-deficient formula. In all cases, blood levels of DHA are higher in babies on either mother's milk or DHA-fortified formula. We can only speculate that these infants have higher DHA levels in their eyes and brains as well.

All of this research indicates the vital importance of the essential fatty acids in the diets of mothers and babies. It is the Omega-3 and Omega-6 fatty acids that build the brain, nerves, and eyes of the baby while it is in the womb, and it is the Omega fats supplied through breast milk that allow the brain to continue to develop after birth. Mothers, take a bow!

CHAPTER 9

THE OMEGA WAY TO MENTAL HEALTH

The Omega fatty acids play a prominent role in a person's mental health. A number of mental disorders, including schizophrenia and manic-depression, may very well be manifestations of an Omega deficiency. In this chapter, we'll first look at some common mental illnesses, and at the connection between the Omega oils and mental health. I'll then provide case histories of some of the twelve patients in my forty-four-patient study who suffered from mental disorders, cases that demonstrate the effects of Omega-3 fatty acids on mental and physical well-being.

Although the patients described in this chapter had been diagnosed with mental illnesses, their reactions to the Omega-oils are relevant to everyone. Nearly all of the forty-four patients in my pilot study reported feeling calmer and less anxious on the Omega Program. Omega oils may do the same thing for you. Of course, if you have experienced some of the symptoms described in the case histories, I recommend that you discuss them with your physician.

THE NATURE OF MENTAL ILLNESS

For many people, affliction with a mental illness is a source of embarrassment in a way that affliction with a physical illness is not. That's because for centuries, mental disorders were ascribed to spiritual or moral defects. However, current research has shown that mental illness commonly arises from physical or biochemical problems that affect the brain.

Today, neuroscience can map the brain with some precision. Physicians can pinpoint which parts of the brain control movement, hearing, sight, and smell, and which parts control emotions, mood, sexual drive, fear, rage, anxiety, and pleasure. The brain's electrical impulses can be recorded as waves on an electroencephalogram (EEG).

Brain disorders are numerous and varied, and depend on which areas of the brain are affected. If motor circuits—the circuits that control motion—are affected, the individual suffers from epilepsy. In epilepsy, abnormal firing of electrical impulses in the brain—a condition noted as extremely rapid brain waves on an EEG—may cause convulsive seizures and unconsciousness. Similar seizures in different brain circuits produce other problems:

- If mood circuits are affected, the individual suffers from manic-depressive disorder, a kind of mood epilepsy. Symptoms vary, from periods of deep depression to periods of intense, abnormal elation. Some people suffer alternating bouts of depression and mania.

- If emotion circuits are affected, the individual suffers

from anxiety attacks, a kind of emotional epilepsy. Symptoms include feelings of overwhelming panic and fear.

- If thought circuits are affected, the individual suffers from schizophrenia, a kind of thought epilepsy. Symptoms include delusions, hallucinations, and psychosis, or detachment from reality.

- If defense circuits are affected, the individual may suffer from agoraphobia—a fear of open spaces—or paranoia—a feeling that one is being persecuted. Both are kinds of defense epilepsies.

And so it goes through the list of mental illnesses.

Because there is a physical cause for so much of mental illness, physicians often prescribe drugs to control symptoms. Lithium is often useful in controlling the mood swings in manic-depression, but relief is often incomplete. For schizophrenic patients, Thorazine and other potent tranquilizers greatly lessen bizarre and psychotic behavior. They do not, however, cure the illness, and many patients find the inertia, drowsiness, and sluggishness caused by these drugs to be intolerable. Undesirable weight gain is another common side effect.

THE OMEGA CONNECTION TO MENTAL HEALTH

As in the case of physical illness, mental illness related to the Omega oils generally has two components: a deficiency in Omega-3 fatty acids, and a deficiency in the vitamins and minerals that allow the body to process the fatty acids.

In fact, mental illness can be seen as part of a group of diet-related illnesses, a group that I have called the modernization-disease syndrome (see Chapter 3). In a susceptible person, the same process that causes spasms in the bowel may trigger spasms of irrational fear, panic, or rage when his or her brain is similarly affected. It may also trigger irrational feelings of euphoria. In a sense, we can view mental illness as an "irritable brain syndrome," a cousin of irritable bowel syndrome and the other irritations caused by dietary deficiencies.

Fatty Acids in the Brain

Essential fatty acids help the brain to function—the normal brain is more than 60 percent fat. Information is transmitted from nerve cell to nerve cell by chemicals called neurotransmitters. The effects of the neurotransmitters are modulated by regulatory chemicals called prostaglandins (see Chapter 2). Disruption of the prostaglandins can cause mental illness.

These prostaglandins are created only from essential fatty acids. As we've seen in previous chapters, if the two main groups of essential fatty acids—the Omega-3 and Omega-6 fats—are out of balance in the diet, proper prostaglandin production is disrupted. When a dietary deficiency of Omega-3 fats destabilizes the production of soothing prostaglandins, there tends to be a buildup of irritating prostaglandins in the brain.

Scientists have found evidence that such imbalances occur in people afflicted with mental illness. The human brain and spinal cord are bathed in nutrient-filled, shock-absorbing cerebrospinal fluid. In people who have schizophrenia, this fluid may contain abnormally low concentrations of certain "good," soothing prostaglandins and abnormally high levels of "bad" prostaglandins—those that constrict blood vessels and cause inflammation. This excess of bad prostaglandins can trigger irritation in brain tissue. But it can be balanced by the calming effects of prostaglandins created from Omega-3 oils.

Many schizophrenics go through periods of severe anxiety before they descend into complete psychosis. During that time, they try to carry on with their lives, although they may feel increasingly fearful. The same progression from anxiety to psychosis takes place in many vitamin-deficiency diseases. Is there a pattern? How does this happen?

It appears that schizophrenia is genetically influenced—it tends to run in families—but is triggered by environmental factors, including dietary ones. The disease often appears during adolescence, a time of growth and hormonal changes that create especially heavy nutrient demands, and often a time of emotional stress and turmoil. Besides subsisting on poor diets, many teenagers and young adults further deplete their nutrient supply by crash dieting in a desperate effort to be fashionably slender. It's a difficult task to get enough Omega-3 in any diet today, and a badly planned diet makes the task impossible.

For a vulnerable youngster with a family history of schizophrenia, obsessive dieting and further reduction of already inadequate amounts of Omega-3 may set the stage for the appearance of psychosis. If sent to a hospital, such patients again live on a diet that is low in fiber and Omega-3 oils. Hospital food is often supplemented by candy, soft drinks, and coffee bought from vending machines. Given the connection between mental health and nutrition, there's reason to be skeptical of chances for improvement in the hospital.

B Vitamins, Prostaglandins, and Your Moods

Obviously, the brain is not exempt from the effects of dietary deficiencies. Heredity probably determines our individual weak spots—how and where the unbalanced or deficient prostaglandins will affect brain circuits that control our thoughts, emotions, moods, and actions. But these weak spots may only give way when nutritional deficiencies strike at the vulnerable centers.

Deficiencies in the Omega-3 fatty acids aren't the only deficiencies that can lead to mental illness. The body needs B vitamins to convert essential fatty acids into prostaglandins. A B-vitamin deficiency can affect prostaglandin production as much as an Omega-3 deficiency. If the body is deficient in Omega-3 essential fatty acids, megadoses of B vitamins may trigger the remaining Omega-3 into action. Although the effect is temporary, the B vitamins appear to neutralize an imbalance of prostaglandins, a task usually accomplished by the missing Omega-3 fatty acids.

MENTAL ILLNESS RESPONDS TO OMEGA THERAPY

Of the twelve mentally ill persons who were part of my forty-four-patient pilot study, what struck me was the number of physical ailments they had. All twelve individuals had many symptoms of modernization-disease syndrome, such as dry skin, fissured fingers, dandruff, arthritis, irritable bowel syndrome, food allergies, headaches, fatigue, and tinnitus. The improvement in seven of these patients' mental illnesses—agoraphobia, mood disorders, and schizophrenia—mirrored unmistakable improvements in their physical condition, and was a direct response to increased levels of Omega-3 in their bodies. Some of the cases discussed in this section also demonstrate the need for careful monitoring and dosage control when using Omega-3 oils to treat serious mental illness.

I observed these individuals at intervals over a one- or two-year period in the early 1980s. Since I was not their primary physician, my contact with them was purposefully kept to the minimum required to monitor progress, or lack of it, in order to eliminate any placebo effect. Afterward, except for unusual developments in the case of

Debi—described later in this chapter—the subjects were lost to follow-up. Other than Debi, all names used are pseudonyms. (For more information on my study, see Chapter 4.)

Agoraphobia

The term *agoraphobia* comes from two Greek words: *phobos*, meaning fear, and *agora*, meaning marketplace or an open place of assembly. In this phobia, certain situations—usually being alone in open or unfamiliar places—trigger such unbearable anxiety and panic that phobics will structure their lives to avoid anxiety-producing circumstances.

Three of the four agoraphobics in my study reacted dramatically to flaxseed-oil supplements. This improvement allowed these people to live fuller, calmer lives.

Kevin, 32 years old, stayed home most of the time. For ten years, it was the only place in which he felt safe. His life was spent avoiding situations that might make him feel anxious. Kevin also suffered from very dry skin on his hands and shins, tinnitus, spastic colon, spasms of the esophagus, poor sleep, and fatigue. The psychiatrists who treated him prescribed a daily dose of Valium, which did not relieve the agoraphobia. They saw no connection between his phobia and his physical complaints.

Two and a half months after he started to take 3 tablespoons of flaxseed oil a day, and while he continued to take the vitamins he usually took, Kevin's skin was healing, he was sleeping better, he hadn't had a single spell of tinnitus or migraine, and his ordinary headaches were less frequent and severe. After a year, all the physical complaints had gotten a lot better, and his anxiety about leaving his house had mostly disappeared.

On two occasions, while visiting relatives a considerable distance from home—in itself an achievement—Kevin went off the flaxseed oil for a week. He told me later that he gradually began to feel tense, but after returning to daily supplements he once again became calm and less agitated.

Marta, 35 years old, had been housebound for eight years. Once or twice a month, she would suffer severe anxiety attacks even without leaving her "safe place." Physically, she had dry skin, dandruff, food allergies, premenstrual syndrome, occasional arthritis, chronic fatigue, and abnormally low blood pressure. One month after starting to take 2 tablespoons of flaxseed oil a day, her hair and skin began to develop a sheen, and she hadn't had a panic attack.

At three months, Marta told me she felt rested and calm, and that she could leave her house, getting as far as the corner without panic. At a year, her physical symptoms had all improved, and her blood pressure had risen close to normal. The areas beyond her home where she now felt safe had expanded considerably.

Chuck was another agoraphobic subject, 58 years of age. He had a long list of chronic physical complaints, including bursitis, tinnitus, dry skin, and fatigue. An active attorney involved in government affairs, he had no problems leaving his home or traveling extensively when his job required it. But for forty years, whenever he crossed an open space—such as a city square—he panicked.

After three months of daily 3-tablespoon doses of flaxseed oil, vitamin supplements, and a fiber-yogurt appetizer, Chuck felt less anxious and was beginning to be able to walk across open spaces. He wasn't sure if all of this was due to the flaxseed oil, or to behavior modification retraining, which he was undergoing at the same time he was taking the supplement. At six months, Chuck reported that his bursitis was much better, his tinnitus was easing up, he wasn't tired all the time, and his skin had some sheen to it.

A year after joining the experiment, Chuck told me he was pretty sure the big drop in anxiety had come from the Omega regimen itself. He still took the flaxseed oil faithfully. It was the ideal backup for the retraining program— Chuck said he was walking confidently across open city areas. He said it helped, though, if he whistled!

My fourth patient had suffered from agoraphobia without letup for twenty years. She was an obese, 53-year-old woman with osteoarthritis, many food allergies, irritable bowel syndrome, and dry skin. She had no response to 3 tablespoons a day of flaxseed oil for two months, except for some softening of dry calluses on her hands. At this point, she dropped out of my study because she was worried about the extra calories from the oil—just at the time when the other agoraphobics were beginning to report improvement.

Mood Disorders

Sadness and feeling "down" are emotions that come and go throughout our lives. But in some people, a crippling despair takes over. Although the initial episode may be triggered by romantic disappointment, financial troubles, or the death of a loved one, the despondency goes well beyond the limits of normal grief. This mood disorder can also appear without any apparently stressful circumstances, leading many experts to conclude there is a physical component to depression.

Unipolar mood disorder describes the major depression that occurs in people who otherwise have normal moods. A *bipolar mood disorder* is one in which periods of inappropriately high elation alternate with periods of deep melancholy. *Manic-depression* is another name for this affliction. The bubbling elation of the manic phase resembles the high of a drug addict. There is a nonstop flight of ideas and activity. The victim feels strong and powerful, but impatience and irritability can lead to an explosive psychotic state.

One of my patients was not helped by flaxseed oil. Sylvia was a 29-year-old woman who had been treated for bipolar mood disorder for a year and a half, and did not respond well to lithium medication. She started on a supplement of 1 tablespoon of flaxseed oil daily, and within six weeks she felt much less tired. There were other physical changes: her color seemed less pallid, and she felt less sensitive to cold.

However, Sylvia then suffered a severe episode of rapid mood swings, from manic elation and agitation to depression. She abandoned the flaxseed-oil supplement, and her physical symptoms returned. She then dropped out of the program. My experience has been that overdosing on flaxseed oil can cause a mood swing in manic-depressives in the direction of agitation and mania. Dosages should be carefully monitored by a qualified professional whenever symptoms of any seriousness are apparent.

Other patients had better responses. Lucy, 32 years old, was diagnosed for twelve years as suffering from paranoid schizophrenia with severe depression. The antipsychotic medication she was given produced side effects—a huge weight gain and reduced thyroid gland function—that required her to take additional medication.

When Lucy was finally put on megavitamins—one gram of niacin three times a day, plus other B vitamins—by an orthomolecular psychiatrist (one who believes that chemical imbalances cause mental illness), she improved so remarkably that she was able to return to work for the first time in many years. However, her daily hallucinations and paranoia continued.

Because of her weight, I started Lucy on 3 tablespoons of flaxseed oil, in doses of 1 tablespoon each, to be taken with her meals. After only four days, she told me her fatigue had disappeared, and she felt elated. She raced through her housekeeping chores, and was once again able to enjoy gardening and other hobbies.

She then increased her dose to a remarkable 9 table-spoons daily, because it elevated her mood. While this erased her schizophrenia, she developed a typical manic attack—the first in her life—which disappeared on stop-ping the oil. Psychological tests confirmed that her real diagnosis was not schizophrenia, but manic-depressive mood disorder. On lithium plus an antidepressant, Lucy felt well and was functioning normally when the pilot study ended.

Hilda was a 43-year-old homemaker and mother who had suffered from unipolar depression for six years. Lith-ium controlled the depression fairly well, but she contin-ued to suffer residual psychosis in the form of sudden violent, murderous thoughts. Physically, Hilda had joint and muscle aches, irritable bowel syndrome, and ex-tremely dry, scaly skin.

After Hilda started taking 3 tablespoons of flaxseed oil a day, the pains eased considerably in just a few weeks. She remained on her usual lithium and thyroid medica-tion. By the seventh week, her scary, violent thoughts were easing, and she felt calm—a feeling she had not enjoyed since the beginning of the psychosis. At four months, hav-ing increased her daily flaxseed-oil dosage from 3 to 5 tablespoons, she had a clear-cut, frightening attack of manic elation, the first in her life. Back on a 3-tablespoon dosage, Hilda's calm returned in a few days. This again demonstrates the need for dosage control.

At seven months, improvement in Hilda's emotional and physical states had accelerated. Her bowel movements became normal, her skin lost its dryness, and for the first winter in memory, she did not develop sore, fissured fin-gers. She also noticed that the unusual thirst she had experienced for many years had disappeared. Although lithium medication can cause thirst, so can an essential fatty acid deficiency. All of Hilda's improvements were holding well when the study ended.

Schizophrenia

The schizophrenic person suffers greatly from bizarre thoughts and distorted perceptions. Hallucinations, weirdly distorted images, or voices are accepted as real. Sometimes, the schizophrenic has lucid moments when he or she realizes that these mental effects are not real.

Ricardo, a 28-year-old paranoid schizophrenic, suffered from bizarre feelings of control. For example, he feared his watching of television news reports would influence world events. Medication partially controlled his psychosis, which had begun eight years before, but his strong paranoid feelings made it uncomfortable for him to be with people. Every night, while trying to fall asleep, Ricardo suffered from what he called his "evening movies"—the hour-long hallucinations that medication couldn't prevent.

After a few weeks on flaxseed oil, at the relatively low dosage of 2 to 4 teaspoons a day, Ricardo's "evening movies" stopped almost entirely. Over the course of the next few months, his sleep improved, his fatigue lifted, and there was a marked decline in his paranoia. Although he still required antipsychotic medication, by the end of the study family members commented on the welcome changes in Ricardo, including his newfound ease and pleasure in the company of others.

Earlier, when I had asked Ricardo to experiment with higher doses of flaxseed oil—6 to 8 teaspoons—he described the beginnings of racing thoughts and feelings of impending psychosis. Dosages for schizophrenics, as for those suffering from mood disorders, have to be monitored carefully by the attending physician. Interestingly, Ricardo lived in a tropical country where, in general, people need less Omega-3 in their diets than people who live in cooler climates. As we saw in Chapter 2, Omega-3 is the cold-climate fatty acid because creatures living in cold places need more of it to keep cell membranes flexible.

Leona was 40 and had been schizophrenic without remission for twenty years. She was under the delusion that she was controlled by invisible wires in her head. Like 90 percent of the pilot study cases, Leona had very dry skin on her hands and flaky dandruff on her shins, for which she used lotion in copious amounts.

Because Leona weighed 200 pounds, I put her on large doses of flaxseed oil: 6 to 9 tablespoons a day. To this, as usual, I added a standard multivitamin supplement. She was in an institution, so she could not improve her diet, and remained on medication.

At two months, the dried, crazed skin on Leona's shins had healed so nicely that she took great pride in showing off her new skin! At four months, however, her mental illness had not gotten better in any visible way. I took her off the program. I suspect now that Leona felt something that her psychiatrist and I could not detect, because months later, when I was in the hospital, she approached me. "Please, doctor," she pleaded, "put me back on the oil! It took the wires out of my head!"

Two other schizophrenic patients in the same institution—who, like Leona, had never shown remission—showed little or no change after a number of months on flaxseed oil. They were less fortunate than the nine other mental patients in my study who experienced regular nonpsychotic interludes during their illnesses. This suggested that improvement was possible on the Omega-3 program.

The most dramatic example of such improvement is Debi Erin (her real name). Debi, aged 26, was my first mentally ill volunteer in my pilot study. She had become schizophrenic at age 16—a time when she was continually crash dieting to become thin. Although she had been hospitalized over and over again, and had been treated by many different specialists, the Debi I saw was still afflicted by daily visual and sometimes auditory hallucinations, intrusive thoughts, and bizarre, sometimes violent, behavior. Her devoted parents had never given up, knowing that their daughter had brief lucid moments each day and was intellectually bright. When conventional treatments failed, her parents had sought out a number of alternative therapies, including megavitamins, food sensitivity testing, and kidney dialysis. Nothing worked for long.

Debi's mother called me after reading an article I had written. Debi describes her pilot-study experience in her own words:

> I must admit at first the whole idea sounded bizarre. Both my mother and I were skeptical. Was this doctor a mad scientist pushing some kind of snake oil? After all the research trials I had been through, surely this was the silliest idea yet.
>
> I tried Dr. Rudin's approach anyway. I took 2 tablespoons of linseed [flaxseed] oil plus a vitamin E supplement. . . . "Oh well, how could it hurt me?" I said to myself. Thirty minutes later, I noticed how calm I was becoming. The sensation of worms in my nerves and quivering in my muscles diminished considerably. After one week on this simple program, my ten-year psychosis subsided. . . . That was in 1980, and I've been free of schizophrenia ever since.

Debi's singular reaction to the oil marked the beginning of a remarkable recovery. After she had gone five months without psychosis, Debi, at my request, cut her daily flaxseed-oil dosage of 4 tablespoons down to 2. Within two days, she had a six-hour psychotic rage! Even after we increased the dosage to 3 tablespoons, she still had trouble sleeping and concentrating. So we went back to the original dosage. At eight months, Debi increased her dosage to 5 tablespoons a day. She began to experience the sensations she used to feel before a psychotic episode—especially the racing thoughts. Again, you should note how important careful dosage control is.

Debi also had a number of physical symptoms, including chronic fatigue, constipation and irritable bowel syndrome, poor sleep, extreme sensitivity to cold, dry skin, and tinnitus in the form of a loud whistling noise. These are symptoms of what I consider to be the modernization-disease syndrome. On the Omega Program, these symptoms abated along with her psychosis. Flaxseed oil, plus supplements of vitamins, minerals, and fiber (see Chapters 11 and 12), gave her relief.

When we ended our contact at three years, Debi no longer needed flaxseed-oil supplements, but remained on the general Omega nutrition program. She didn't need antipsychotic medication, either. And she was going to college; when I reestablished contact with her, I found she was working as a registered nurse in a psychiatric hospital.

THE MENTAL-HEALTH BENEFITS
OF THE OMEGA PROGRAM

The cases described in this chapter are different in many ways, but a single thread runs through them: in at least seven out of twelve patients, Omega-3 fatty acids produced improved behavior, contributed to feelings of well-being, and reduced psychotic thinking. Also, a great many of the mentally ill patients also experienced a lessening of their physical problems—irritable bowel syndrome, joint diseases, tinnitus, food allergies. Thus, there are many possible benefits from Omega-oil supplementation, including greater peace of mind.

The results of my study found acceptance among physicians who had long believed there was a connection between nutrition and mental health. In the 1950s, psychiatrists Abram Hoffer and Humphrey Osmond pioneered the use of nutritional therapy, combined with medical treatment, for schizophrenics and other mental patients. Later, this combined treatment became known as orthomolecular psychiatry. The term "orthomolecular" was devised in 1968 by Linus Pauling, who suggested that in order to restore balance to the body, we must supply it with the "right molecules" in the form of vitamins, minerals, and other nutrients. From long experience, Hoffer and Osmond found orthomolecular psychiatry to be more effective than conventional treatment alone in righting the chemical imbalance within the brain that produces schizophrenic symptoms.

In the early 1980s, after journal articles on my study appeared, Hoffer and other orthomolecular practitioners began observing benefits in patients who were given Omega-3 oils, in addition to their other supplements, for the first time. In 1995, after he had treated twenty-six chronic mental patients for ten years or more, Hoffer wrote about the results of their treatment. One patient had not improved at all, five were improved, three were much improved, and *eighteen* were well and functioning successfully in the outside world—compared with what may be only 5 *percent* significant recovery among patients in conventional psychiatric treatment. Hoffer is convinced that orthomolecular psychiatry will eventually become standard practice.

If you would like to feel calmer and more in control of your life, then the Omega Program—described in Chapters

11 and 12—may be for you. But as we've seen, people with severe mental illness have to take carefully controlled dosages of any medication, whether it be flaxseed oil or a standard prescription medicine. Therefore, if you have been diagnosed with, or think you may suffer from, a mental illness, please see your physician before starting any supplement program.

CHAPTER 10

THE OMEGA
ANTIAGING BENEFITS

We tend to think of death as the ultimate end of every living thing. But most one-celled life forms—bacteria, yeast, algae, and protozoa—never die of old age. They live forever, ceaselessly dividing, unless stopped by predators, starvation, or accidents.

However, multicelled life forms, up to and including humans, are genetically programed to age and die. Let's take a look at how aging takes place, and at how it is tied to nutrition. We'll then see what you can do to fight the aging process.

AGING AND OUR IMMORTALITY GENE

The outward signs of aging are obvious to everyone: graying hair, wrinkles, age spots, slower movements, and so on. They are especially irksome when we notice them in ourselves! These outward signs reflect internal changes, changes that start in the individual cell. As our cells age, the tissues and organs made up of the affected cells begin to decline in function.

This decline shows up in the ailments and disorders we associate with age, such as heart disease, arthritis, and diabetes. Other diseases, such as cancer, result from a less-efficient immune system, which can no longer keep mutant cells in check. Still other diseases, such as pneumonia, result from the immune system's inability to rid the body of viruses and bacteria. While these conditions do occur in younger people, they tend to be more serious in the elderly.

What happens to our cells that causes them to age? Cells contain genes, the carriers of our inherited traits. Genes direct the production of all protein enzymes—chemicals that direct all bodily processes—in our cells and organs. As time goes on, our genes are exposed to a variety of harmful factors. Some of these factors, such as chemical pollutants and radiation, enter the body from the outside. Other factors, such as harmful cell-function byproducts called free radicals, attack the body from the inside. Eventually, more and more of our genetic material is damaged, and the cells' ability to make vital enzymes is compromised.

But the one-celled organisms that can live forever, and the multicelled organisms that cannot survive indefinitely, share an "immortality gene." This gene produces a specific enzyme that repairs genetic damage before it can turn into cell damage. Just as the body's immune system destroys abnormal cells, so the enzyme produced by the immortality gene destroys deviant gene copies, and repairs or replaces genetic material.

Why then, in spite of our hardworking immortality gene, are we and all other multicelled life *not* immortal? The cause may be a biological time bomb—some scientists call it the "death gene." Theory has it that when the right time arrives for each species, the death gene becomes acti-vated and begins to suppress the immortality gene. By blocking the immortality gene's repair work, the actions of the death gene gradually lead to a buildup of faulty gene copies. These, in turn, either produce faulty enzymes or shut off production of some enzymes altogether. Enzymes are involved in *thousands* of ongoing functions in every cell of the body. Sooner or later, defective or missing enzymes will cause these functions to slow down. Thus, the death gene, by obstructing the priceless repair work of the im-mortality gene, sets the stage—cell by cell—for aging and, in the long run, death.

We can learn about the behavior of the genetic-repair system by looking at diseases that involve damage to the genes. One of these diseases is cancer. When normal cells are transformed into cancer cells, they behave like one-celled life forms and keep reproducing themselves. They no longer respond to the body's essential fat-prostaglandin regulatory system, described in Chapter 2, which "civilizes" all of the body's cells and keeps them working together as a unit.

Two other diseases that involve genetic damage are rare disorders that produce the full range of aging problems in early childhood. In the diseases progeria and xeroderma pigmentosa, the afflicted children—who often die before they reach their teens—look wizened and old, and suffer baldness, dry skin, age spots, arthritis, heart disease, and strokes. A deficiency of the gene-repairing enzyme, the one produced by the immortality gene, is involved in these ailments. It's as if the death gene had switched off the immortality gene some seventy years too soon!

Because the aging process involves the deterioration or loss of many enzymes, it will affect the way the body handles essential fatty acids and prostaglandins. This regulatory system needs specific enzymes to do its impor-tant work. The ailments seen in children suffering from progeria and xeroderma pigmentosa look very much like the disorders caused by failing essential fatty acid-prostaglandin controls.

I saw many signs of what looked like premature aging among the volunteers in my forty-four-patient study (Chapter 4), even though these people were in early middle age or younger. After I gave them the Omega-3 fatty acids they were missing, the volunteers and I saw welcome changes in their dry, rough skin, sallow complexions, age spots, glaucoma, and arthritis. The big surge in Omega-3 studies, which began in the 1980s, is providing more and more evidence that these oils may also reduce rates of heart disease and cancer (see Chapter 5).

NUTRITIONAL ANTIAGING FACTORS

The concept of defective gene repair as being the key to aging is well accepted. It has been hard, however, to identify the specific gene system, enzymes, or nutrition patterns that speed up the aging process, despite numerous attempts to do so. Too much sugar, saturated fat, and trans-fatty acids are on the list of prime suspects. Many studies focus on the bad consequences of eating too little fiber. Others single out free-radical damage to cells as a major accelerator of aging. And some scientists say that too much Omega-6 and too little Omega-3 in the diet are doing us in too soon.

My own conclusion is that, together, all of these elements derail the major director of cell activity—the essential fatty acid-prostaglandin regulatory system. In fact, I suspect that this system may be the prime target of the death gene! Enzymes that process the Omega-6 and Omega-3 fats in the body are known to decline with age. And as we've seen, many of the disorders associated with aging are hard to tell from disorders caused by a fatty acid-prostaglandin imbalance.

To prevent premature aging, which actually appears to be more like an aging disease, we must do everything we can to protect and tone up our fatty acid-prostaglandin system. Such efforts may also slow down what is now considered to be the normal rate of aging.

Aging experiments that involve humans are impractical because our potential life span is so long—close to 110 years. But some hints come from animal studies. For instance, when rats were given antioxidant supplements that protect essential fats in tissues from free-radical damage, the rats lived longer. These antioxidants—selenium and vitamin E—protect against free-radical damage in our bodies. In another example, a breed of short-lived mice survived much longer when given fish-oil supplements containing the Omega-3 fat EPA. And in yet another example, mice given all the required nutrients, but kept systematically underfed, have survived about 50 percent longer than their usual life span. Underfeeding apparently stimulates a key enzyme that processes the body's essential fats, an enzyme whose activity tends to decline with age. I suspect, though, that the prospect of remaining half-starved in order to live longer has little appeal for most of us!

Malnutrition Leads to Aging

Two kinds of malnutrition exist—dietary and metabolic. *Dietary malnutrition* occurs when there is a lack of nutrients in the diet. In dietary malnutrition, levels of nutrients in the bloodstream are usually low. *Metabolic malnutrition* occurs when nutrients are in the diet, but the body's ability to use them is impaired. In metabolic malnutrition, nutrient levels in the bloodstream may be normal or even high. But the nutrients don't reach the cells, so the tissues are starved.

It is this second type of malnutrition that comes into play as the body ages, since aging tends to slow down the body's ability to process nutrients. At the same time, the deficiencies of the modern diet promote dietary malnutrition. Therefore, older people tend to be in a double-jeopardy situation: they don't get enough of the nutrients they need, and they can't use the nutrients they do get very efficiently. Unfortunately, these two forms of malnutrition tend to feed off of and aggravate each other, thus begetting a vicious circle. It becomes easy for the older person to become very malnourished.

Aging also brings a declining requirement for calories, since an older body is generally a slower body that doesn't use as much energy as it did when it was younger. But when calorie needs fall below 1,500 calories a day, it becomes very difficult to obtain even a minimum daily requirement of various nutrients from food alone.

In either situation—malnutrition caused by diet or malnutrition caused by metabolism—supplements should be used. Supplements can not only provide the nutrients that are not provided by the diet, but can provide them in sufficient quantities to overcome many of the problems the body may have in using nutrients properly.

Ways to Fight the March of Time

Most of us would like to fight the effects that age has on our bodies, and many of us go to great lengths in order to do so. But an antiaging regimen does not have to be either time-consuming or expensive. Here are four ways to help fight the aging process:

- Make sure you get enough Omega-3 oil. Increase your fish consumption to at least one serving a week. Older people may benefit especially from fish-oil supplements containing the Omega-3 ultrapolyunsaturates EPA and DHA. Also supplement your diet with flaxseed oil. See

Chapters 11 and 12 for supplementation guidelines provided by the Omega Program.

- Take a complete multivitamin and multimineral supplement every day. This supplement should include the antioxidants—beta-carotene, vitamin C, vitamin E, and selenium—in addition to the other vitamins and minerals discussed in Chapter 11.

- Make sure you eat enough fiber—have a fiber appetizer (see page 149) before breakfast, lunch, and dinner. Fiber not only prevents constipation, but it can also help clear out unneeded cholesterol from the body (see Chapter 3). Use flaxseed or flaxseed meal as a source of both the anticancer fiber called lignan and the essential fatty acids.

- Participate in a program of aerobic exercise suitable to your strength and health. Aerobic exercises, which strengthen the heart and lungs, include walking, jogging, and cycling.

Within these guidelines, try eating different ratios of protein, carbohydrate, and fat over a three-week period. Note your reactions by keeping a food diary—it will help you find your optimum diet. (If you believe you may have food allergies, see "Testing for Food Allergies" on page 155). High-protein meals are often used as supplemental diets before surgery or to give debilitated people a boost. Avoid high-protein diets, however, if you have liver or kidney disease, because the body's processing of proteins places an additional burden on these organs.

SHEDDING THE BURDENS OF AGE

Among long-vanished preindustrial—so-called "primitive"—societies, the elders were valued teachers of tribal history and customs, passing along the lore that a tribe needed to ensure its survival. Modern-day elders not only provide their families with a sense of history and continuity, but are being called on, more and more, to take on active roles in the community. Seniors are teaching, writing, acting in movies and television, doing volunteer work, and serving as political movers and shakers. Remember, we're living longer now, and staying younger—and not because of face-lifts!

Can we live forever? Probably not any time soon, if at all. But our longevity depends on the amount of gene-repairing enzyme our bodies make, the enzyme that is under the control of the immortality gene. When this gene is shut off by the death gene, we know we're on the downward slope.

We've seen that cancer cells, although usually nipped in the bud by an alert immune system, are, in theory, immortal. They divide and grow like one-celled life forms, no longer fazed by the death gene. But one organism doesn't have to contract cancer to nullify its death gene. A primitive multicelled fungus called *Neurospora* can, depending on environmental conditions, shift from its usual state, in which it ages and dies in a few months, to an immortal state. This takes just a few genetic mutations, after which *Neurospora* can go on forever—at least in principle. Given the ease with which our cells can become immortal by turning into cancer cells, scientists suspect that we, too, carry genes that can switch off the death gene.

In the meantime, the Omega Program, described in Chapters 11 and 12, is our best bet for staying healthy. Good health will be more important than ever if the genetic engineers figure out how to make us immortal!

CHAPTER 11

THE OMEGA PROGRAM–
PHASES 1 AND 2

The Omega Program is the first supplementation program to be designed around the
Omega-3 essential fatty acids—the "good
fats" the body needs to function properly. When the
Omega-3 fats provide the missing link, a powerful new
teamwork becomes possible among the remaining nutrients. This directly benefits the body.

I recommend the Omega Program for everyone who has
subsisted on a modern diet, even if they feel healthy. Remember, some conditions, such as atherosclerosis and diabetes, may develop for years before you notice symptoms.
But I especially recommend the Omega Program for those
who are not in good health.

I'll explain the first two phases of the Omega Program
in this chapter, and the second two in the next. Take a
minute to read "Consult Your Physician First" on page 137.

PHASE 1: SELECTING AND ADJUSTING YOUR OMEGA-3 OIL INTAKE

In this section, I'll first help you decide what oil is best, and how you should buy and store it. I'll then explain how to find the dosage that's right for you.

What Kind of Oil Is Best?

As we've seen, the modern diet does not contain balanced amounts of the two groups of essential fatty acids—the Omega-3 and the Omega-6 oils. We tend to eat a lot of the Omega-6 oils, which come from plants that grow in southern climes, and not enough Omega-3 oils, which come from plants and animals in northern climates (see Chapter 2).

Therefore, I suggest using only nonhydrogenated northern oils. These are flaxseed oil, walnut oil, wheat germ oil, and soybean oil; see Table A.1 for the Omega-3 contents of these oils. All southern oils—such as corn, cottonseed, olive, sesame, peanut, or safflower oil—have very little Omega-3.

Flaxseed oil, with its high Omega-3 content, is the best supplement oil. It is mild tasting, relatively inexpensive, and very safe. Most important, it works. Although the long-term effects of flaxseed-oil supplements have not been determined, flaxseed oil itself has been used as a food oil for thousands of years. It is a first cousin to the cod-liver oil supplements of yesteryear.

You can fulfill part of your Omega-oil requirements from the foods you eat. Easy-to-find food sources of Omega-3 are fatty fish (such as mackerel and salmon), soybeans, wheat germ, chestnuts, and walnuts (see Table A.2).

Flaxseed oil, and many other oils, are available from most health food stores, either in large capsules or in small capsules called perles. Twelve large (1 gram) capsules equal

Consult Your Physician First

If you suffer from a serious health problem, or if you are planning to have a child, consult your physician or nutritionist before starting the Omega Program—especially if you are planning on trying fairly high dosages of anything. He or she will tell you what I'll tell you: start low and gradually work your way up.

Secretions of the skin and other organs are often normalized on the Omega Program. Preexisting cystic conditions may clear up, or plugged ducts in the skin, ovaries, or elsewhere may spontaneously open, making surgical relief unnecessary. However, these conditions may worsen if the cyst outlets remain completely blocked and secretions increase. In that case, only you can judge if the benefits warrant continuing the program.

about 1 tablespoon of flaxseed oil. Five perles equal one large capsule.

Why start the Omega Program with plant-based oil instead of fish oil, and why flaxseed oil instead of the other oils that contain Omega-3? Flaxseed oil contains ALA, the first fatty acid in the Omega-3 family. The body cannot make ALA, but can transform it into EPA and DHA, the Omega-3 fats found in fish oils. ALA also has a special effect in directing the kinds of prostaglandins the body makes. And, as we've seen, flaxseed oil is safe.

Buying and Storing Your Oil

Here's the first step in the program. Besides using the flaxseed oil for both cooking and supplementation, use only nonhydrogenated soybean, walnut, or wheat germ oils for cooking, along with small amounts of butter. *Throw out* all other salad and cooking oils. Also consign to the trash *all* solid shortenings, hydrogenated lard, and solid margarines. They are loaded with harmful trans-fatty acids (also known as trans fats), the fatty-acid imposters that insinuate their way into cell membranes and compete with the good fats (see Chapter 2). Trans-fatty acids are bad news for health!

The flaxseed oil suggested for use in the Omega Program is food-grade oil. *Do not* confuse food-grade flaxseed oil with boiled linseed oil from paint and hardware stores. Nutritional flaxseed oil is available in health food stores in most areas. If your store doesn't carry it, ask them to order it for you. It is also listed in most health-food catalogs.

Ideally, whatever oil you use should be cold pressed. Cold-pressed oils are produced by putting mechanical pressure on batches of seeds. In this method, heat-producing friction is low and temperatures remain below 110°F during pressing and any subsequent refining process. Health-food stores carry cold-pressed, unrefined flaxseed oil.

Try to get the oil in dark glass containers that are sealed airtight. Examine the label and avoid a product that is partially or lightly hydrogenated. Smell, then taste, all oils before using them to be sure they are not rancid. The flavor should be nutty to slightly fishy, and always fresh tasting.

To avoid rancidity, buy oil in pint quantities and use each bottle within a few months after opening. Refrigerate the oil as soon as the bottle is unsealed—it should keep well in the refrigerator. Without refrigeration, it quickly becomes rancid after opening. Extra oil can be stored in the freezer; it won't freeze, but it will stay fresher longer.

Some people fear that flaxseed oil becomes rancid too rapidly. But in my experience—confirmed by that of colleagues, patients, and friends, and backed up by laboratory tests—is that the danger of instant rancidity is highly exaggerated. Remember, this oil has been used as a kitchen oil for thousands of years.

Finding and Taking the Right Dosage

How nice it would be if I could tailor a program with just the right dosage of Omega-3 oils to suit everyone! That's impossible, unfortunately, because each of us has a different need.

The effectiveness of each oil can vary, so you must experiment, preferably starting with flaxseed oil. The minimum daily flaxseed-oil requirement for any adult eating 2,000 calories a day is 1/2 teaspoon. If you take any less, do not expect any therapeutic benefit.

My recommended daily allowance for most adults who are not suffering any overt Omega-3 deficiency symptoms is 1 teaspoon. However, those who suffer ailments related to an Omega-3 deficiency may find they need much more than 1 teaspoon for a period of months. Here are guidelines for daily megadoses of flaxseed oil, developed from my pilot study (see Chapter 4):

Body Weight (pounds)	Dosages (all approximate)
100	1 tablespoon
125	1 to 2 tablespoons
150	2 to 3 tablespoons
175	3 tablespoons
200	3 to 4 tablespoons

A dosage of 1 to 4 tablespoons (12 to 48 one-gram capsules) was needed daily for the first few months by most of the people in my pilot study. Only by constantly monitoring, adjusting, and experimenting could we determine each person's optimal dose. Likewise, you must be prepared to develop your own program. Increase your dosage gradually every few days.

If there is any chance that you might be sensitive or allergic to oil—for instance, if you already have allergies—start with 1 teaspoon (approximately four capsules) a day, and increase that dose gradually every four days. (If you think you may have a food allergy, see "Testing for Food Allergies" on page 153.) Remember, it may take a while to experience the desired benefits. Don't randomly increase dosages just because you aren't getting immediate results. And if you are increasing a dosage, stop if a side effect develops (see "Avoid Excessive Meganutrients" on page 141). Also, you should note that 1 tablespoon has approximately 100 calories, so you should cut calories elsewhere if you are concerned about weight gain.

In my study, patients very often discovered a threshold dose was needed to achieve a therapeutic effect. For instance, there might be no tangible result from 1 teaspoon of flaxseed oil taken daily over many weeks or months. However, with an increase in dosage from 1 to 2 teaspoons, there would be a complete remission of symptoms—of osteoarthritis, for example—in a few weeks.

Flaxseed oil should be taken, in divided doses, with meals whenever possible, instead of all at once. Some people take it neat, others prefer to follow the oil with orange juice. Capsules or perles of flaxseed oil may be more convenient. To make the large capsules easy to swallow, soften them in warm water for a few minutes before attempting to swallow them. You can also stir flaxseed oil into soups or other liquid foods, or it can be used in salad dressings.

If you suffer from gallbladder or digestive problems related to fat metabolism, taking two or three soy lecithin capsules along with the flaxseed oil may help. The lecithin can help emulsify the oil, allowing it to be absorbed with less discomfort.

PHASE 2: ADDING THE COFACTORS—
VITAMINS, MINERALS, AND FIBER

The Omega-3 nutrients are probably not the only nutrients

Avoid Excessive Meganutrients

Meganutrients can interact. I do not recommend taking limitless amounts of any nutritional supplement, because nutrients in very large amounts can, like anything else, have adverse effects, and this is especially true if you are taking megadoses of several nutrients at once. The most common negative result of megadoses is to reintroduce the original illness that the nutrients were originally taken to alleviate.

Start with a vitamin supplement that provides only the Recommended Dietary Allowance (RDA) of each vitamin and mineral, and increase only one group of vitamins at a time. Be alert to any changes in your bodily functions. If adverse effects appear, lower the dose or stop for a few days, then start again at a lower level.

How do you know when you are taking too much? It is a good idea to note any changes in your mood, skin, or stamina on a daily basis. If your skin is dry, you should check it daily. When your dosage is adjusted correctly, your skin will develop a soft, slight sheen a few weeks after starting on the program—provided, of course, the rest of your nutrition is adequate.

You can continue to increase your flaxseed-oil or other essential nutrient intake gradually, in three-day increments. But stop if you notice any adverse effects, such as bloating, gas, dizziness, headache, diarrhea, sleepiness, or muscle aches. Bear in mind, however, that the safety margin for flaxseed-oil therapy is high compared to that of most medications and drugs. It would take about ten times the therapeutic dose for any toxic symptoms to appear. In general, I would recommend that you do not take dosages greater than those recommended in the Omega Program without talking to your doctor or nutritionist.

There are some other guidelines to keep in mind. Too much whole flaxseed or flaxseed meal can produce a vitamin B6 deficiency. More than 50,000 IU a day of vitamin D for several

months can cause dizziness, diarrhea, nausea, fatigue, and kidney stones. Too much iron, copper, or zinc can block the absorption of other minerals.
   All of these effects are rare in people who eat sensibly. When
they do occur, they are usually reversible and are mild in comparison to the extremely dangerous side effects produced by conventional drugs.

missing from your diet. Vitamins, minerals, and fiber are
also lacking in the average American diet. But the body
works by cooperative efforts. Certain enzymes—chemicals that direct all bodily processes—are needed to convert the Omega fats into prostaglandins. These enzymes,
in turn, need B vitamins and minerals to help promote
transformations in the Omega fats. As these highly unsaturated fats become part of our tissues, they must be
protected from free-radical oxidation—a kind of rust, or
rancidity, if you will. Antioxidant vitamins and minerals
defend fatty acids against this damage. And fiber coop-
erates with the Omega fats to help keep blood-cholesterol levels normal.

   To achieve the optimum results from your Omega Program, it is necessary to add these cofactors. You must
overcome all deficiencies—bring yourself to a normal
level—before you can see the greatest therapeutic benefit.
You must also reduce the antinutrients, such as white
flour, refined sugar, and hydrogenated and trans fat, in
your system. As I said in Chapter 3, antinutrients inhibit
or alter the actions of nutrients needed for proper bodily
functioning.

   For the fastest results, undertake Phases 1 and 2 at the
same time. Some people prefer to delay the start of Phase
2 so they can track their progress on the oil supplement

alone. In any case, you should start Phase 2 within three or four weeks of beginning Phase 1. Keep in mind that the oil and the cofactors multiply each other's actions, and that this can lead to side effects—see "Avoid Excessive Meganutrients" on page 141.

The Vitamin Cofactors

The Omega-3 vitamin cofactors are vitamin A, the B vitamins, vitamin C, and vitamin E.

Vitamin A

What and Why. Vitamin A is an antioxidant that works with vitamins C and E, and with the mineral selenium, to protect the essential fatty acids. The health of the skin and mucous membranes throughout the body depends on a diet that is adequate in vitamin A. Vitamin A is also essential for normal vision and healthy teeth, gums, and sex glands. A lack of vitamin A will show up in dry, scaly skin and visual problems. Also, cancers of the gastrointestinal tract and lungs have been produced in animals deficient in this vitamin.

How Much and Food Sources. There are two ways to get vitamin A. You can get it directly, in foods of animal origin, such as liver or eggs. Or you can get it in the form of beta-carotene (also known as pro-vitamin A), which comes only from plants. There is no evidence of problems resulting from the consumption of foods containing large amounts of beta-carotene, from which the body makes its own vitamin A. However, you can get too much vitamin A from fish-liver oils, so keep cod-liver oil intake down to 1 teaspoon daily.

Some people who eat large amounts of carotene-containing foods—oranges, carrots, dark leafy vegetables, and deeply colored fruits—have noticed that their skin seems to turn yellowish. I recommend taking 10,000 IUs of beta-carotene and never more than 20,000 units, especially when on high oil dosages. In supplement form, be very wary of vitamin A—25,000 to 50,000 IUs a day can result in toxicity symptoms within a few months. These symptoms include headaches, fainting, nausea, joint pains, diarrhea, and skin problems. If you are planning a pregnancy, or if you are pregnant, you shouldn't take more than 8,000 IUs a day of vitamin A.

The B Vitamins

What and Why. The B vitamins boost the action of the Omega-3 fatty acids. If you now take B vitamins, either in a daily multivitamin or in a B-complex supplement, you may find you must reduce your present dosage as your Omega-3 deficiency is overcome. The beneficial effects you previously felt from vitamin B supplements may have come about, in part, because of their effect on the Omega-3 fatty acids in your body.

Vitamin B_6 appears to play a pivotal role in making prostaglandins, the regulatory chemicals described in Chapter 2. Supplements in amounts considerably over the RDA have had beneficial effects on diseases similar to some of the Omega-3 deficiency diseases—arthritis, premenstrual tension, and heart disease.

How Much and Food Sources. If you've never taken vitamin supplements, begin with the major B vitamins—see Table 11.1. Start at the lowest level and gradually work up to a level that relieves your symptoms (see Table 12.1 for an idea of when you might expect to see results). Once your condition improves and stabilizes, retest by using smaller and smaller dosages as the months go by, until you find the lowest

Table 11.1. Megadoses of B Vitamins

Vitamin	RDA	Recommended Range
B$_1$—thiamin	1.5 mg[1]	5 to 6 mg
B$_2$—riboflavin	1.7 mg	5 to 7 mg
B$_3$—niacin[2]	19 mg	50 to 100 mg
B$_5$—pantothenic acid	7 mg	25 to 50 mg
B$_6$—pyridoxine	2 mg	6 to 8 mg
B$_{12}$—cyanocobalamin	2 mcg[3]	25 to 50 mcg
Biotin	0.1 mg	0.2 to 0.5 mg
Folacin—folic acid	0.2 mg	0.5 to 1 mg

1. "mg" stands for "milligrams."
2. Most people will feel a niacin flush—a flushing and tingling of the face and ears for a few minutes—after taking 50 to 200 mg of niacin.
3. "mcg" stands for "micrograms."

dosages that give you optimum results. The major B vitamins have been used in high doses for long periods of time with a good safety record. Side effects are unusual. Stopping the dosage reverses any side effects in nearly all cases.

Good sources of various B vitamins are yeast, wheat germ, liver, legumes, milk, nuts, seeds, eggs, and fish.

Vitamin C

What and Why. Vitamin C is a potent antioxidant that protects tissues from damage. However, controversy rages over the amount to be taken in supplement form. The RDA is set at about 60 milligrams for adults, but some scientists feel that high intake can be useful in combatting cancer, the common cold, hepatitis, and other viral disorders. There are also studies indicating that it can lower blood cholesterol.

How Much and Food Sources. For people without kidney problems, I see no danger in starting at 500 milligrams of vitamin C and gradually increasing the daily dosage to between 1 and 2 grams. Amounts greater than that can cause diarrhea and flatulence. In rare cases, large over-doses can contribute to the development of kidney and bladder stones, but adequate supplementation with vitamin B_6 and magnesium can usually prevent this problem. Good food sources of vitamin C include broccoli, Brussels sprouts, horseradish, kale, sweet peppers, cabbage, cauliflower, chives, spinach, and strawberries.

Vitamin E

What and Why. Vitamin E is another important antioxidant that protects the essential fatty acids within our bodies. As we increase our Omega-3 intake, our tissues will reflect this in increased levels of polyunsaturated fats. These tissues will need extra protection against rancidity. As a sensible precaution, vitamin E supplements should be taken along with other antioxidants—beta-carotene, vitamins A and C, and selenium—because they interact to guard our tissues. A 1996 study in Cambridge, England, which involved more than 2,000 people with heart disease, showed that high doses of vitamin E (400 or 800 IU) substantially reduced the incidence of heart attack over a two-year period.

How Much and Food Sources. I recommend taking 50 to 250 IUs of vitamin E a day. Amounts up to 800 units daily over long periods of time have been proven safe in major studies. One physician reported problems with blood clots in heart patients who had regularly taken high doses of vitamin E, but this has not been seen in large trials with the vitamin.

Foods rich in vitamin E include wheat germ, oatmeal, avocado, green leafy vegetables, berries, and sweet potatoes. Seeds and nuts that contain unsaturated oils often are good sources of vitamin E.

The Mineral Cofactors

Calcium and selenium are the major mineral cofactors, along with several trace minerals.

Calcium

What and Why. Calcium is the most abundant mineral in the body, and it is responsible for many vital functions. The importance of maintaining the strength of bones and teeth is obvious: low calcium is linked with osteoporosis. Also, when in proper balance with other minerals—sodium, potassium, magnesium, and phosphorus—calcium helps regulate the rhythmic contractions of the heart and other muscles. It also stabilizes nerve conduction.

How Much and Food Sources. It is generally recognized that only about 30 percent of the calcium you eat daily is actually absorbed. Not enough dietary magnesium, too much coffee or tea, the use of laxatives, or the consumption of large amounts of protein can interfere with calcium absorption.

A reasonable adult calcium dosage is about 1,200 milligrams a day. Because this amount of calcium cannot be fitted into a multivitamin and multimineral supplement pill, you must take calcium supplements separately. Calcium citrate is better absorbed than most other calcium compounds.

Dairy foods are good sources of calcium, as are salmon, sardines, and green, leafy vegetables such as turnip greens.

Selenium

What and Why. The trace mineral selenium appears to have a special role in guarding the good fats in cell membranes. A lack of this mineral in the soil of certain parts of Canada and the United States means that crops grown in this soil don't provide enough selenium for our needs.

How Much and Food Sources. The RDA is set tentatively at 50 to 200 micrograms; I recommend a supplement of from 5 to 25 micrograms if taken in the chelate form, which is easier for the body to absorb. Determine your own tolerance level. Amounts of 500 mcg or more can cause garlic breath, eczema, and neurological problems.

Fin fish, shellfish, and animal or poultry liver (and other organ meats) are reliable sources of selenium.

Other Essential Trace Minerals

What and Why. Copper, zinc, and manganese are other important antioxidants. These are trace minerals, which means you only need very small amounts of any of them. (The amino acids methionine and cysteine are also antioxidants, and are found in protein foods.)

How Much and Food Sources. Because these minerals are needed in such small amounts, the toxic levels of most trace elements are very close to the required level. Some of these minerals are very potent, even in very small amounts. In addition, large doses of one mineral may suppress absorption of other nutrients. For example, a very high copper intake—more than 20 milligrams per day— has been found to interfere with zinc absorption. So take care with mineral supplements.

Copper is found in a wide variety of foods. Zinc is found in seafood, meats, poultry, whole grains, and legumes. Manganese is found in nuts, seeds, whole grains, and avocados.

The Fiber Cofactor

Fiber is an important part of your diet. The foods that sustained our ancestors were high in fiber. But today's processed food is scant in both Omega-3 essential fatty acids and fiber. We generally only get 10 grams of fiber a day, compared with the recommended amount of 25 to 35 grams. Although fiber is not yet officially considered an essential nutrient, even conservative doctors are hinting at a connection between serious ailments and fiber deficiency.

To make sure you get the fiber you need, eat a diet with a lot of fruits and vegetables, whole grains, and legumes. See Table A.3 for the fiber contents of various foods.

As part of the Omega Program, I recommend that you have a fiber-yogurt appetizer before every meal (see page 150). This appetizer contains both soluble and insoluble fiber: the former reduces blood-cholesterol levels, the latter improves bowel movements. Within two or three days after you start taking the appetizer, it should produce odorless, coil-shaped bowel movements. If your stool is poorly formed, reduce the amount of fiber at each meal by about 1/4 tablespoon.

You might feel bloated or gassy for about a week after you start the fiber supplement. That's because the bacteria in your digestive tract need some time to adjust to the presence of extra fiber.

Once you start taking fiber on a regular basis, constipation should not be a problem. If it is, use a vegetable-based laxative for a short period of time. But do not use laxatives regularly without consulting your physician.

If you travel a great deal, there are fiber supplements well suited to your needs. You can get fiber tablets that contain both soluble and insoluble fiber. You can also eat commercially prepared fiber-yogurt bars.

Getting Fiber Into Your Diet

For a quick, high-fiber snack, you can combine fiber and yogurt. Mix 1 tablespoon of bran or 1 teaspoon of flaxseed meal with 1 tablespoon pectin or 1 teaspoon psyllium powder into 2 tablespoons of yogurt. Or you can use 1 tablespoon bran plus 1 teaspoon each of pectin and psyllium. Or, use one of these recipes.

Mixed Bulk Fiber

28 servings

2 cups (4 ounces) miller's bran or oat bran, or 1 cup (2 ounces) flaxseed meal

¼ cup (1 ounce) psyllium seed powder

1 tablespoon (¼ ounce) pectin powder (optional)

Mix the ingredients together in a jar. Cover and store, dry and sealed, in a cool place or the refrigerator. To use, add 1 rounded tablespoon of the mixture to yogurt and water (see the Fiber Appetizer recipe). You can also add ¼ teaspoon wheat germ to each serving, if you wish.

Fiber Appetizer

1 serving

1 tablespoon miller's bran or oat bran, or 1 teaspoon flaxseed meal

¼ teaspoon psyllium seed powder

2 tablespoons plain yogurt

¼ teaspoon wheat germ (optional)

1 to 2 tablespoons water or juice

Combine all the ingredients in a wide-mouthed glass. Mix together lightly, adding water or juice to desired consistency. Wait a few minutes for mixture to soften before eating. Follow it with a glass of water.

Note: if you are allergic to milk, substitute low-sugar applesauce for the yogurt, or take acidophilus capsules instead. If you have colitis, start with small amounts and work up to the suggested amount.

CHAPTER 12

THE OMEGA PROGRAM–
PHASES 3 AND 4

In Chapter 11, we covered the first two phases of the Omega Program—choosing and using your Omega-3 oil, and using the Omega cofactors (vitamins, minerals, and fiber). In this chapter, I'll explain Phases 3 and 4. Phase 3 is the maintenance phase, in which you'll learn how to taper your supplements back to a maintenance level after your Omega-3 deficiency symptoms have eased. Phase 4 is the balancing phase, in which you'll learn how to balance your Omega-oil intake.

PHASE 3: MAINTAINING THE PROGRAM

Now that you've been on the Omega Program awhile, the next step is to monitor yourself and evaluate your response to the program. This step is important because the addition of the Omega-3 fats means you are now on the first nutritionally complete supplement program. The combined effects of the supplements will be greatly enhanced by the Omega-3. For this reason, you are especially susceptible to the toxic effects of meganutrients.

The goal is always to take the minimum amounts of supplements needed to correct a condition or illness, and then to cut back to a maintenance level after a time, letting the Omega Program carry you. After all, on this program you will be getting probably five to ten times the Omega-3 of your previous diet, even after you taper off.

It is important to make sure you don't have any food allergies that may be acting as hidden impediments to good health—see "Testing for Food Allergies" on page 153. It is also important to remember that you must exercise and reduce your stress levels to make the Omega Program work—see "Increasing Exercise and Decreasing Stress" on page 161.

In this section, we'll see how your skin will tell you whether or not the program is working for you. We'll also see how you can cut the amounts of both your oil supplement and your cofactor supplements back to maintenance levels.

The Skin as a Window on Health

Your skin is a window on your internal well-being. I find skin response a convenient guide for discovering what levels of Omega-3 flaxseed oil and what cofactors work best for most patients. Working together, we often adjust the flaxseed-oil dose to get a visible reduction in skin dryness, generally in about three to four weeks. The resulting smoothing of the skin, added sheen to the hair, and brightening of the eyes are delightful to see, and are sure evidence that something good is happening throughout the body.

Many people with very dry skin on their hands, feet, and other body parts have, ironically, excessive oil on their forehead, eyebrows, scalp, and nose. The oil from overac-

Testing for Food Allergies

Many of the people who participated in my forty-four-patient study suffered from immune-system problems, including food allergies. These allergies revealed themselves in symptoms such as diarrhea, breathing difficulties, hives, nausea, quickened heartbeat, headaches, and a flushed feeling. These symptoms occurred within a few hours after eating the offending food or foods. However, when the symptoms were not violent, many of the victims did not realize that they had suffered allergic reactions, since these foods were eaten so regularly that their correlation with illness was difficult to trace. Keeping a food diary—a written account of exactly what has been eaten for several days— and noting daily symptoms can sometimes uncover the troublemakers. Another common approach is to see an allergy specialist for a lengthy and expensive series of tests.

I suggest following the Omega Program to see if that eliminates the problem over a period of several months. If it doesn't, your immune system may be so overwhelmed by food allergens that you cannot respond to any therapy until the allergens have been identified and removed from your diet. To find out what foods are causing your reaction, first try the Omega food elimination diet. If that doesn't help you find the problem, try the Omega chemical sensitivity diet.

THE OMEGA FOOD ELIMINATION DIET

Food allergens are everywhere. The most common food allergens include:

Beans	*Fish*	*Peas*
Chocolate	*Garlic*	*Shellfish*
Citrus fruits	*Milk*	*Tomatoes*
Corn	*Nuts*	*Wheat*
Eggs	*Onions*	*Yeast*

Many people are also sensitive to a number of food additives:

• *Monosodium glutamate (MSG)—often used in Chinese cooking and in prepared foods*

• *Nitrates and nitrites—found in luncheon meats, hot dogs, ham, and bacon*

• *Sulfites—used to keep greens fresh, and sometimes added to vegetables in salad bars*

Products that contain one or more of these ingredients, even in small quantities, can cause all sorts of allergic reactions, from wheezing to rashes. People with arthritis tend to be sensitive to foods in the nightshade family, such as tomatoes, eggplant, peppers, and potatoes, all of which contain solanine, a steroidlike compound.

To identify the offending food or substance, the common allergens previously listed, along with any other suspected foods, must be eliminated from the diet for a period of two weeks. Instead, follow Diet No. 1 in the accompanying chart. If no improvement occurs after two weeks on Diet No. 1, try Diet No. 2 for two weeks. If still no improvement occurs, try Diet No. 3. You should see improvement on one of these three diets. If not, try Diet No. 4, which is a milk-only diet.

Follow each diet strictly. This means no restaurant meals, since you cannot determine exactly what ingredients are being used. It also means carefully reading food labels. For example, ordinary rye bread contains some wheat flour, and the elimination diets specify no wheat whatsoever.

When you find a diet that relieves your symptoms, start adding foods from the allergen list, one at a time, back to your diet in large amounts for at least three days to see which foods provoke an adverse reaction.

This procedure will detect allergies to milk and gluten, a protein found in all cereals. Both are very common allergies that can cause skin rashes and gastrointestinal discomfort. I think another form of this allergy may be a major contributor to mental illness. If such allergies are discovered, a gluten- or gluten-and-milk-free diet is recommended. You may find that after several months on the Omega Program, your allergy disappears as your immune system returns to normal. However, allergy management can be a complex issue, so do not try any diet without first discussing it with your physician.

THE OMEGA CHEMICAL SENSITIVITY DIET

For some people, following the food elimination diet may not uncover the offending foods. In such cases, the most effective dietary method for detecting a food allergy is to use a chemical liquid diet in which all food components are reduced to their elemental, nonallergic nutritive forms. This is the diet used to prepare people for gastrointestinal surgery, and is related to liquid weight-loss diets. Many people have lived for a number of years sustained by such diets alone.

Such liquid diets are available through pharmacists without prescription; one commercially available diet is Vivonex. However, as with any other diet, you should only use a liquid diet under the guidance of a physician.

The liquid diet should be fortified with an oil rich in Omega-3, about 1 to 3 tablespoons for every 2,000 calories of liquid drink. The diet should also be supplemented with fiber. However, you should first test for possible allergic factors in the oil and fiber themselves. To do so:

1. *Start with the liquid diet alone for a week.*

2. *On the eighth day, add an Omega oil, either soybean, walnut, or flaxseed oil. Switch to a different oil every five days, and note any reactions, negative or positive, that may occur.*

3. *After cycling through all three oils, introduce fiber—either pectin, psyllium seed, or miller's bran. Switch to another fiber every five days, and note any reactions, negative or positive, that may occur. Keep the oil constant while cycling through the fibers.*

If you find yourself feeling frustrated with your lack of progress, see your doctor or nutritionist. If improvement is noted, reduce the liquid diet by half and eat foods from a specific food group in either of Diets 1, 2, or 3. If you experience a reaction to a particular food or food group, go directly to a numbered diet that does not contain the suspect food or foods. Your symptoms should abate. You can then guess which food causes your allergic reaction. As a double check, eat the suspect food and see if that provokes a reaction.

Food Allergy Elimination Diets

Foodstuff	Diet No. 1 No beef, pork, fowl, rye, corn, wheat, or milk	Diet No. 2 No beef, lamb, rice, wheat, or milk	Diet No. 3 No lamb, fowl, rye, rice, corn, wheat, or milk
NOTE: Diet No. 4 consists solely of milk.			
Cereal	rice products	corn products	none
Vegetables	lettuce, beets, spinach, artichokes, carrots	corn, tomatoes, peas, squash, asparagus, string beans	lima beans, string beans, tomatoes, potatoes (white and sweet)
Meat	lamb	chicken, ham	beef, bacon
Flour	rice	corn, 100% rye (ordinary rye contains wheat)	lima bean, soybean, potato
Fruit	lemons, pears, grapefruit	peaches, prunes, apricots, pineapple	grapefruit, peaches, lemons, apricots
Fat	walnut oil	flaxseed oil	soybean oil
Beverage	tea, lemonade, black coffee	spring water	juice from approved fruits, black coffee, tea
Misc.	tapioca, cane sugar, gelatin, olives, salt	corn syrup, gelatin, salt	tapioca, honey, gelatin, olives, salt
Milk	none	none	none

Source: Adapted from *The Merck Manual*, sixteenth edition (Rahway, NJ: Merck Research Laboratories, 1992).

tive sebaceous glands causes greasy scales and dandruff. This problem is called seborrheic dermatitis, and is related to an Omega-3 deficiency. Seborrheic dermatitis tends to normalize on the Omega Program. As the hands and feet become smoother and softer, the skin of the scalp is freed from scales. Once my patients find the flaxseed-oil and cofactor dosages that produce the best results for them, they stay on their own personal programs for at least two or three months, or until their skin shows substantial improvement.

Depending on your health circumstances, it may be several days to a week or several months before you see definable improvement (see Table 12.1). In unusual cases, the response can be immediate. Once you recognize improvement, continue on your supplementation program for a year or more, but during this time, try gradually decreasing dosages as low as you can without again incurring trouble.

Continue on any existing medication that has been prescribed by your physician. Try to avoid over-the-counter medications. As time goes by, you may find that your need for medication, and for megadose levels of supplements, decreases dramatically. When this happens, if you continue on the original prescription or continue to take the same amount of vitamin supplements, you may develop toxic side effects (see "Avoid Excessive Meganutrients" on page 141). As your need for medicine, drugs, or vitamin supplements decreases, you should reduce the amount you take of each proportionally. You are your own best guide, but you should consult your physician.

Adjustments and Maintenance

It is not always easy to find your optimum supplement level. In my Omega-3 pilot study, when we were unable to

Table 12.1 When to Expect Benefits
from the Omega Program

These response times come from the Omega-3 pilot study that I did in the early 1980s (and which is described in Chapter 4). The response time varies with the symptom experienced. In some cases, improvement can continue for up to one or two years before leveling off. Allergies often require a long time. Nothing is guaranteed, because each person's makeup is so different. Persistent emotional or physical problems may improve only after several months—if at all.

Time After Starting Oil Supplement	Reaction
2 hours	Mood is improved Depression is lifted
2 to 7 days	Skin becomes smooth, with less flaking and scaling
2 to 14 days	Fewer hallucinations among mental patients Anxious feelings are relieved
2 to 6 weeks	Osteoarthritis is improved, with easier movement and less pain Bursitis and other soft-tissue inflammations are reduced Tinnitus and other ear noises subside Dandruff and scalp flaking are less noticeable, dry skin is alleviated
2 to 4 months	Rheumatoid arthritis pain is diminished Easy bruising is reduced Fewer muscular spasms Choking spells subside Fewer nighttime leg cramps Ocular spasms (eye cramps) are reduced Itching and burning of the skin are relieved Skin color is improved Sun sensitivity is reduced
3 to 6 months	Food allergies (see page 153) are diminished Chronic infections are healed Rough, bumpy skin on upper arms becomes smooth Alcohol tolerance is improved Cold tolerance is improved Fatigue is lessened Feelings of calm and well-being are increased

achieve a positive change, I suspected the cause to be one of the following:

- Too little flaxseed oil—the oil dosage was increased

- Cofactor deficiency—the vitamin dosage was increased

- Cofactor excess, such as too high an intake of B vitamins or vitamin A—the vitamin dosage was decreased

There are other reasons why the program may not work initially. It may be that your body cannot convert the primary Omega-3 fatty acid, ALA, into the longer-chain Omega-3s, EPA and DHA. This may require the use of fish oil instead of flaxseed oil, because fish oil contains ready-made EPA and DHA (see page 163). Or, perhaps, your body is not absorbing the nutrients properly.

No matter why you think you're not responding, I would suggest that you talk to your physician or nutritionist. He or she can do the sorts of tests that can help you find your proper dosage.

After the pilot-study volunteers had been on the Omega Program for three months, I asked them to reduce their intake of flaxseed oil by half for a few weeks while keeping the cofactors steady, and other fats and oils in the diet as low as practical. If previous problems did not recur and no new problems manifested themselves, the patients were asked to reduce the dose by half again. This dosage lowering continued until the original symptoms reappeared. In this way, each individual could stabilize at the lowest effective dose of flaxseed oil. Another way to lower the Omega-3 dosage is to switch to supplements of walnut or soy oil, which have a lower Omega-3 fatty acid content.

After a few weeks, while holding the oil level steady, my patients reduced their supplemental vitamin and mineral doses by half for a few days, or a week, and carefully noted the response. Again, this is the way to find the lowest effective dosage. Every few months, my patients used this same technique to recheck both the oil and cofactor dosages. As long-term healing took place, the requirements for oil, vitamins, and minerals often declined.

It is important for you to find the lowest effective dose as you continue on the program. The original dose can be too strong for a long-term program. A dosage level that helped you originally actually may cause a toxic reaction later on. (Some medications may do the same thing.) A very few subjects in the pilot study still required 3 tablespoons of flaxseed oil daily after two years on the diet. But for most, the requirements dropped drastically—usually from one to six months after starting the program. The benefits of the Omega Program were greatest by then, too.

PHASE 4: BALANCING THE OMEGA-3
AND OMEGA-6 FATTY ACID GROUPS

The final phase of the Omega Program—balancing your flaxseed-oil level with the levels of other oils—completes the picture. This final stage of fine-tuning requires that you gradually explore the optimum ratio of different oils in your diet. See Table A.1 for a listing of the fatty-acid contents of various oils.

Some Final Notes on Flaxseed Oil

One patient in my Omega-3 study reported that applying flaxseed oil to the skin of her varicose veins reduced the pain that had been brought on by walking. Other subjects have noticed that arthritis and eczema improve with local application of flaxseed oil. However, I have also seen irritations result from applying flaxseed oil to seborrheic dermatitis of the face and scalp. If you are considering external

Increasing Exercise and Decreasing Stress

Too little exercise builds up stress, and can undo a lot of the good done by eating a proper diet. Exercise and stress reduction are important parts of the Omega Program.

Exercise does a lot of good things for your body. It:

- *Strengthens the heart, lungs, and bones*
- *Improves intestinal function*
- *Improves mental outlook*
- *Allows you to eat more food without gaining weight*

There are two main forms of exercise, aerobic and anaerobic. Anaerobic exercise, such as weightlifting, can increase your muscle mass, but aerobic exercise can help you live a longer, healthier life because aerobic exercise improves the body's use of oxygen. I recommend that you get thirty minutes' worth of aerobic exercise three times a week. While such activities as basketball and running are good forms of aerobic exercise, you certainly don't have to push yourself at that pace. A good, vigorous walk is fine, or you can jog (outdoors, or indoors on a small trampoline) or ride a bicycle.

Stress reduction, like exercise, can help both your body and your mind. There is no way to measure stress—until you suffer the results. But you can take measures to avoid stress:

- *Exercise.*
- *Meditate. If you have troubles you can't deal with by yourself, seek counseling.*
- *Find an enjoyable job. Workplace pressures are stressful for many people.*
- *Get one hug a day. (This is my minimum daily requirement. The RDA is two hugs, and three or more hugs a day is the therapeutic megadose!)*

application of flaxseed oil, a good precaution is to test a small, dime-sized area of skin for at least forty-eight hours before applying it to a wider area.

Remember that if you are taking flaxseed oil—or any supplemental oil, for that matter—it is very important to take the vitamin and mineral cofactors, especially selenium. If you are deficient in this important antioxidant mineral, an intake of supplemental essential fatty acids may only make the selenium deficiency worse. Whatever selenium stores are in your body will be used up that much sooner in an attempt to protect the essential fatty acids from oxidation. This means that Omega Program oils may make health symptoms worse over a period of weeks and months *unless* sufficient vitamin, mineral, and fiber cofactors are available on a regular basis.

It is also very important to remember that too much oil can cause your original symptoms to reappear. I have learned through experience that if there is a toxic effect— such as dry skin or mental confusion—it generally means that the person has simply "turned up the dial" too much. Gradually balancing the amounts of oil and cofactor supplements restores the previous gains and brings the patient back to comfortable health.

There's one more thing you should know about using flaxseed oil. Flaxseed, along with such drugs as ibuprofen, aspirin, and cortisone, all have an effect on prostaglandin production. And each has side effects:

- Excessive aspirin or ibuprofen use can cause tinnitus, stomach damage, and reduced kidney function.

- Excessive cortisone use can cause severe muscle soreness, stomach ulcers, swelling of the extremities, and many other disorders.

- Excessive flaxseed oil and excessively large amounts of

vitamin supplements can cause tinnitus, muscle soreness, and other problems. However, the safety margin
for flaxseed oil is quite high. It would take about ten
times the therapeutic dose before toxic symptoms might
appear.

Anyone taking prescription medications should discuss
possible medication side effects with his or her physician,
or check the *Physicians' Desk Reference* (known as the PDR,
often available in local libraries). You should avoid over-
the-counter medications. If you do take them, be alert to
changes in your total health. If any symptoms of drug
toxicity appear after you start the Omega Program, find
out if a lowered dose of medication is feasible. If it is not,
then lower the flaxseed-oil dose.

Balancing with Fish Oils

If, after a few months on flaxseed oil, you feel the need for
further improvement, you may want to explore the benefits to be derived from fish oils. These oils will provide you
with EPA and DHA, the long-chain Omega-3 fatty acids
that are not present in flaxseed oil. It may be that your body
is not able to create enough of these fats from ALA, the
primary Omega-3 in flaxseed oil.

EPA is needed to create "good," or healing, prostaglandins that are beneficial to the cardiovascular system and cell
membranes throughout the body. DHA is vital for a
healthy brain, and for healthy eyes and sex organs.

Begin by reducing your daily flaxseed-oil dosage by
half, and adding from one third to one half the maximum
dose—1 teaspoon—of fish oil. Adjust gradually, every
week or so, until you find the optimum amount. Do *not*
exceed 1 teaspoon of cod-liver oil, the most commonly
used fish oil. Remember, vitamin A can build up to toxic

levels in the body's fatty tissues, and cod-liver oil contains a lot of vitamin A. You may also use up to six capsules of fish-oil concentrates such as Maxepa or Promega each day.

A combination of fish and vegetable oils may be most effective in slowing down the production of "bad" pro-staglandins—those responsible for menstrual cramps and for feelings of emotional turmoil—and encouraging the "good" prostaglandins—those that enable cells to heal and provide a feeling of calm and well-being. (Prostaglandins are discussed in detail in Chapter 2.)

Balancing with the Omega-6 Oils

Remember, if you live in a cold climate, you need higher amounts of Omega-3 oils. The Omega-3 essential fatty acids provide cell membranes and tissues with extra flexi-bility, something that is otherwise reduced in cold weather. That's why plants and animals that live in cold climates, and fish that live in colder waters, contain more Omega-3 in the first place. Conversely, if you live in a warm climate, you may need less Omega-3, because your body doesn't have to withstand severe cold. This need may, however, depend as much on your inherited traits as it does on the climate in which you live.

Start by substituting about half the flaxseed oil you have been taking with safflower oil, which has a high ratio of Omega-6 to Omega-3—between 58 and 75 percent to only about 1 percent. Continue to increase the safflower oil and decrease the flaxseed oil until you see a change in your skin or general health.

An alternative method is to switch to walnut or soy oil, which have a lower ratio of Omega-3 to Omega-6 fatty acids—10 percent to 40 percent—than flaxseed oil. You must be alert for any change in your health, for better or worse. Keep asking yourself, "Is my skin getting softer and smoother? Do I feel better or not?" As Richard Kunin, noted nutrition author says, "Listen to your body."

This continued experimentation and evaluation will guide you in working out an optimum ratio of Omega-3 to Omega-6 oils—and the minimum supplement amount—that is best for you. Recheck in this manner every few months to keep your oil dosages in balance.

Another way to balance the Omega-3 and Omega-6 oils in your diet is to take evening primrose oil, which is high in Omega-6 gamma linolenic acid (GLA). GLA can sometimes mimic and augment the effects of Omega-3 oils inside the body. Capsules of evening primrose oil can be bought in health food or drug stores—a reliable brand is Efamol.

Start with capsules supplying about 40 to 80 milligrams of GLA a day and work up to 240 to 320 milligrams a day. British researcher David Horrobin and other scientists report numerous therapeutic benefits of this Omega-6 oil. Like the Omega-3 oils, evening primrose oil can direct the activity of the "good" prostaglandins, the ones that promote soothing and healing.

Several of my patients have found that taking evening primrose oil alone aggravated their health problems, but that it was helpful when combined with flaxseed oil and fish oil. Only testing will tell what balance works best for you.

FOLLOWING THE OMEGA PROGRAM FOR BETTER HEALTH

The Omega Program was designed for those who suffer from specific physical or mental health problems, especially symptoms of the modernization-disease syndrome. It is also good for those who just want to feel better. This program can also improve stamina for people whose zest for life outstrips their ability to keep going to the end of the day.

The four phases of the Omega Program—choosing the

Omega-3 oil and dosage, adding the cofactors, tapering back to a maintenance program, and balancing the oils—may seem a little complicated at first. But I can assure you that, in practice, it is fairly simple, and will soon become a part of your daily routine. A few minutes a day—plus time for proper exercise—can add up to a lifetime of health.

Don't get trapped in expensive supplement programs. The Omega Program should cost you no more than from a few pennies to fifty cents a day, unless you need very large amounts of expensive fish oils and megavitamins for a short period of time. Work out your own optimum dosage for the various nutrients, following the guidelines in this book. Shop for your supplies at your local nutrition store, at the nutrition center in your supermarket, or via mail order from nutrition supplement catalogs.

I have observed how well—one might say how grate-fully—the body responds *at any age* to removal of antinu-trients and replacement of needed substances, especially the "missing link" fatty acids. Respect your untapped capacity for repair and renewal, and anticipate a payoff of better health and well-being.

I hope the Omega Program works for you.

APPENDIX A

SOURCES OF OMEGA FATTY ACIDS AND FIBER

Table A.1. Oil Sources of Fatty Acids

Selected fatty-acid contents of various oils are given as grams per 100 grams of oil (approximately 3 ½ ounces). All data are for nonhydrogenated oils. This table has been compiled from many scientific sources; values may vary with season, temperature, and nutrient source.

Grams per 100-gram portion (approximately 3½ ounces)

Sources	Omega-6 EFA[1] Linoleic	Omega-3 EFA Alpha linolenic	EPA	DHA	Total EFA	Total fat content
FISH OIL						
Cod, Atlantic	1.2	0.8	12.4	21.9	41.7	100
Halibut, Pacific	0.9	0.3	10.1	7.9	26.9	100
Mackerel	1.1	1.3	7.1	10.8	29.3	100
Rockfish	1.6	0.8	11.7	17.4	36.1	100
Salmon, Chinook	1.1	0.9	8.2	5.9	20.6	100

Sources	Omega-6 EFA[1] Linoleic	Omega-3 EFA			Total EFA	Total fat content)
		Alpha linolenic	EPA	DHA		
Salmon, coho	1.2	0.6	12.0	13.8	33.6	100
Sole, lemon	0.7	2.0	14.7	6.8	36.6	100
Tuna, albacore	0.7	0.6	6.5	17.6	25.4	100
Tuna, bluefin	1.3	TR[2]	6.6	20.8	28.7	100
FISH LIVER OIL						
Cod, Atlantic[3]	1.5	0.9	8.0	14.3	29.7	100
SHELLFISH OIL						
Oyster, Pacific	1.2	1.6	21.5	20.2	51.7	100
Scallop, sea	0.6	0.3	21.3	26.2	55.7	100
VEGETABLE OIL, Omega-6 sources— tropical to temperate climates						
Cashew	16	0.4	0	0	16	100
Coconut	3	N/A[4]	0	0	3	100
Corn	57	0.8	0	0	58	100
Cottonseed	48	0.4	0	0	48	100
Evening primrose[5]	72	0.2	0	0	81	100
Olive	9	0.7	0	0	10	100
Peanut	29	1.1	0	0	30	100
Poppy seed	69	N/A	0	0	69	100
Pumpkin seed	51	N/A	0	0	51	100
Safflower	58	N/A	0	0	58	100
Sesame	42	0.5	0	0	42	100
Sunflower	53	N/A	0	0	46	100
VEGETABLE OIL, Omega-3 sources— temperate to polar climates						
Canola (rapeseed)	22	11	0	0	33	100
Chestnuts, European	35	4	0	0	39	100
Flaxseed (linseed)	15	55	0	0	63	100
Hempseed	62	19	0	0	81	100
Perilla	16	67	0	0	83	100
Soybean	53	7	0	0	60	100
Walnut	67	4	0	0	71	100
Walnut, black	62	7	0	0	69	100
Walnut, English	55	11	0	0	66	100
Wheat germ	54	7	0	0	61	100

Sources	Omega-6 EFA[1] Linoleic	Omega-3 EFA			Total EFA	Total fat content)
		Alpha linolenic	EPA	DHA		
ANIMAL FAT						
Beef tallow	4	0.7	N/A	N/A	4.2	100
Butter	1.8	1.2	N/A	N/A	3.0	80
Chicken fat	17	1.1	N/A	N/A	17.6	100
Lard	10	1.4	N/A	N/A	11.8	100
Mutton fat	5	2.9	N/A	N/A	8.1	100

1. EFA = essential fatty acids. Total EFA includes these listed plus others, if any are not listed here.
2. TR = trace.
3. Toxic at high dosages.
4. N/A = not available in sources checked.
5. Contains 8.6 grams of Omega-6 gamma linolenic acid (GLA).

Table A.2. Food Sources of Omega Fatty Acids

Selected fatty-acid contents of various foods are given as grams per 100 grams (approximately 3 ½ ounces) of food. All figures are for raw food, unless cooked is specified. This table has been compiled from many scientific sources; values may vary with season, temperature, and nutrient source.

Grams per 100-gram portion (approximately 3½ ounces)

Sources	Omega-6 EFA[1] Linoleic	Omega-3 EFA			Total EFA	Total fat content
		Alpha linolenic	EPA	DHA		
DAIRY PRODUCTS						
Cheeses, natural						
Cheddar	0.5	0.4	N/A[2]	N/A	0.9	33
cream	0.8	0.5	N/A	N/A	1.3	34
Gouda	0.3	0.4	N/A	N/A	0.7	27
Gruyère	1.3	0.4	N/A	N/A	1.7	32
Roquefort	0.7	0.8	N/A	N/A	1.5	34
Cheeses, processed						
American	0.6	0.3	N/A	N/A	0.9	29
Cheddar	0.7	0.4	N/A	N/A	1.1	30
Cream						
heavy	0.9	0.6	N/A	N/A	1.5	38
light	0.5	0.3	N/A	N/A	0.8	21
sour	0.4	0.3	N/A	N/A	0.7	18
Desserts						
ice cream,						
vanilla	0.8	0.2	N/A	N/A	0.5	12
pudding,						
tapioca	0.3	0.1	N/A	N/A	0.4	5
Milk, cow's	0.1	0.1	N/A	N/A	0.2	4
FOWL, roasted						
Chicken						
dark meat	1.9	0.1	N/A	0.1	2.4	9.7
light meat	1.3	0.1	N/A	0.1	1.6	6.4
Turkey						
dark meat	1.1	0.1	N/A	0.2	1.5	5.3
light meat	0.5	0.03	N/A	0.1	0.7	2.6
EGG YOLK, chicken, hard-boiled (approx. 4 yolks)						
Supermarket						
eggs	2.6	0.05	N/A	0.1	3.6	23
Flaxmeal eggs[3]	4.2	2.1	0.05	0.5	7.4	26

Sources	Omega-6 EFA[1] Linoleic	Omega-3 EFA			Total EFA	Total fat content
		Alpha linolenic	EPA	DHA		
KERNELS, NUTS, AND SEEDS, Omega-6 sources— tropical to temperate climates						
Cashews	7.3	0.2	0	0	7.5	46
Coconut flesh	0.7	0.0	0	0	0.7	36
Corn	28.5	0.5	0	0	29.0	50
Cottonseed	11.5	0.1	0	0	11.6	23
Olive	5.6	0.5	0	0	6.1	68
Peanut	14.4	0.6	0	0	15.0	50
Poppy seed	32.0	N/A	0	0	32.0	47
Pumpkin seed	17.0	N/A	0	0	17.0	33
Safflower	20.0	N/A	0	0	20.0	35
Sesame	19.2	0.2	0	0	19.2	48
Sunflower	12.0	N/A	0	0	12.0	27
KERNELS, NUTS, AND SEEDS, Omega-3 sources— temperate to polar climates						
Chestnut	0.9	0.1	0	0	1.1	3
Flaxseed (linseed)	7	17	0	0	24	38
Perilla	6	27	0	0	33	40
Soybean	11	2	0	0	13	21
Walnut, Black	37	4	0	0	41	60
Walnut, English	35	7	0	0	42	63
Wheat germ	6	0.7	0	0	7	11
MEAT						
Beef, broiled						
Steak, average of flank or sirloin	0.3	0.1	N/A	N/A	0.4	7.5
Ground, 77% lean	0.5	0.3	N/A	N/A	0.9	21.2
Lamb, roasted or broiled						
Loin, 66% lean	1.2	0.6	N/A	N/A	1.9	32.4
Leg, 82% lean	0.8	0.3	N/A	N/A	1.2	21.2
Rib, 62% lean	1.4	0.7	N/A	N/A	2.1	36.0
Organ meats						
Beef heart, lean, cooked	0.7	0.01	N/A	N/A	1.1	0.7
Beef liver, lean, cooked	1.1	0.1	N/A	N/A	1.5	10.6

Sources	Omega-6 EFA[1] Linoleic	Omega-3 EFA			Total EFA	Total fat content
		Alpha linolenic	EPA	DHA		
Pork liver, cooked	1.3	0.1	N/A	N/A	1.8	11.5
Pork						
Ham, roasted or broiled, 84% lean	1.8	0.2	N/A	N/A	2.1	19.6
Spareribs, braised	3.5	0.3	N/A	N/A	4.2	39.0
Bacon, smoked, cooked	4.7	0.6	N/A	N/A	5.4	49.0
Luncheon meat, canned	3.1	0.4	N/A	N/A	3.6	30.1
Sausage, cooked	3.4	0.4	N/A	N/A	3.9	32.5
Sausages, pork and beef						
Bologna	1.7	0.3	N/A	N/A	2.1	27.5
Frankfurter	2.4	0.4	N/A	N/A	2.9	28.9
Vienna sausage	1.6	0.3	N/A	N/A	2.0	25.2
Veal loin, roasted, 85% lean	0.6	0.2	N/A	N/A	0.9	13.6
MILK, HUMAN						
Australia	0.4	0.02	0.01	0.01	0.5	4
North America	0.6	0.04	0	0.01	0.73	4
Malaysia	0.4	0.01	N/A	0.04	0.46	4
SEAFOOD						
Fin fish, fillets						
Cod, Atlantic	N/A	N/A	0.08	0.15	0.26	0.7
Flounder	0.01	0.01	0.11	0.11	0.35	1.2
Halibut, Atlantic	N/A	N/A	0.10	0.30	0.43	1.1
Halibut, Greenland	0.07	0.02	0.27	0.22	0.73	8.4
Halibut, Pacific	0.02	0.03	0.11	0.20	0.55	2.0
Herring, Atlantic	0.29	0.11	0.33	0.58	1.43	6.2
Herring, Pacific	0.12	0.03	0.76	0.57	1.67	11.1
Mackerel, Atlantic	0.14	0.10	0.65	1.10	2.44	9.8
Rockfish	0.04	0.02	0.32	0.48	0.98	3.1

Sources	Omega-6 EFA[1] Linoleic	Omega-3 EFA			Total EFA	Total fat content
		Alpha linolenic	EPA	DHA		
Salmon, Atlantic	0.08	0.05	0.18	0.13	0.51	5.8
Salmon, Chinook	0.13	0.11	1.0	0.72	2.49	13.2
Salmon, coho, Pacific	0.08	0.04	0.82	0.94	2.28	7.5
Salmon, sockeye— canned	0.15	0.41	0.62	1.0	3.44	6.7
Salmon, sockeye— fresh	1.40	0.31	1.30	1.70	4.71	8.9
Sole, lemon	N/A	N/A	0.09	0.09	0.27	0.8
Tuna, albacore— canned	0.05	0.04	0.38	1.10	1.81	6.8
Tuna, bluefin— canned	0.03	0.02	0.33	0.63	1.17	4.6
Shellfish						
Crab, Alaska King, legs and claws, cooked	0.03	0.04	0.33	0.15	0.62	1.6
Clam, flesh	0.03	0.02	0.08	0.07	0.28	1.4
Oyster, Pacific, flesh	0.03	0.04	0.42	0.29	0.90	2.3
Scallop, different species, flesh	0.01	N/A	0.12	0.14	0.35	0.91
Shrimp, different species, flesh	0.02	0.01	0.18	0.15	0.47	1.2
Snail, pond, flesh	0.10	0.09	N/A	0.36	1.14	2.80
Spiny lobster, Caribbean, flesh	0.03	0.01	0.18	0.09	0.59	1.2
SEEDS, LEGUMINOUS						
Bean, dried— kidney, navy, pinto, red	0.3	0.6	0	0	0.9	1.5
Broad bean	0.7	0.1	0	0	0.8	1.6
Chickpea	2.2	0.1	0	0	2.3	5.0
Cowpea	0.5	0.3	0	0	0.8	2.0
Garden pea, green	0.3	0.1	0	0	0.4	0.8

Sources	Omega-6 EFA[1] Linoleic	Omega-3 EFA			Total EFA	Total fat content
		Alpha linolenic	EPA	DHA		
Lentil	0.4	0.1	0	0	0.5	1.2
Lima bean	0.4	0.2	0	0	0.7	1.4

1. EFA = essential fatty acids.
2. N/A = not available in sources checked.
3. When flaxmeal is added to feed, hens' eggs contain more Omega-3.

Table A.3. Dietary Fiber Amounts of Various Foods

Food	Amount	Dietary Fiber (grams)
BREADS		
Bread, white	1 slice	less than 1
Bread, whole wheat	1 slice	1 to 2
Graham cracker	2	0.5
Rye wafer	2	2
CEREALS		
All-Bran	1/3 cup	8.5
Bran flakes	3/4 cup	4
Corn flakes	1 cup	0.5
Corn grits, cooked	1/2 cup	0.3
Oatmeal, cooked	3/4 cup	1.6
Puffed wheat	1 cup	0.5
FIBER SUPPLEMENTS		
Flaxseed meal	1 rounded teaspoon	1
Miller's bran	1 tablespoon	4
Oat bran	1 tablespoon	2.5 to 3
Psyllium fiber	1 teaspoon	3
FRUITS		
Apples	1 medium	4
Bananas	1 large	3
Blackberries	1/2 cup	3
Blueberries	1/2 cup	2
Cantaloupe	1/4 melon	1
Grapefruit	1/2 medium	2
Grapes	20	0.5
Peaches	1 medium	2
Prunes	3 medium	3
Raspberries	1/2 cup	3
Strawberries	1 cup	3
NUTS		
Almonds	10	3
Brazil nuts	10	5
Filberts	10	1
Peanuts	10	1.4
VEGETABLES AND LEGUMES		
Broccoli, cooked	1/2 cup	2
Cabbage, cooked	1/2 cup	1
Carrots, cooked	1/2 cup	2
Celery, raw	1/2 cup	1
Corn, cooked	1/2 cup	3

Food	Amount	Dietary Fiber (grams)
Lentils, cooked	1/2 cup	4
Lettuce	1 cup	1
Navy beans, cooked	1/2 cup	6
Peas, cooked	1/2 cup	4
Potatoes, with skin	1 medium	2.5
Spinach, cooked	1/2 cup	2
Tomatoes, raw	1 large	2

A NOTE TO PHYSICIANS

A s I mentioned in the text of this book, the evidence indicates that the bulk of illness in modern societies is the result of an un-recognized disease cluster that I call the modernization-disease syndrome. This cluster is caused by a multitude of food and dietary modifications interacting metabolically with stress and exercise deficiency. The food modifications have never been tested for their collective safety by health authorities, and it seems clear that they interact in the body to produce a new kind of deadly synergistic malnutrition that is not caused by any one factor alone. The resulting biochemical disturbances center on a newly discovered fat-based regulatory system—the essential fatty acid-pro-staglandin system—that regulates just about every body function. These disturbances, when playing against ge-netic variations, can then cause just about every illness known to medicine.

This modernization-disease syndrome is the fatty cousin of the classical B-vitamin deficiency diseases of pellagra and beriberi. These diseases were the result of food modifications, many of which continue to this day, and to which we have added many others. Now we are succumbing to similar problems all over again, and for the same reason. The ultimate cause is a persisting structural defect in our health-care delivery system and health-care regulation that tolerates a medical monopoly, even though our primary health problems are not medical but are instead related to nutrition and lifestyle. The result has been to put the health of our entire society at risk for the second time in the past 100 years.

As a researcher for thirty-five years, first in the Neurophysiology Laboratory of Anesthesiology at Massachusetts General Hospital (within the Department of Pharmacology at Harvard Medical School) and later as Director of the Department of Molecular Biology in a clinical setting at the Eastern Pennsylvania Psychiatric Institute in Philadelphia, I wondered if ignorance of the chemistry and nutrition of lipids—one of the last great biochemical families to be worked out—might prevent us from recognizing a lipid deficiency/toxicity syndrome in humans. After all, deficiencies or excesses of every other major nutrient family—proteins, minerals, vitamins, and fiber—have been identified, after lengthy scientific investigations, as major public health hazards, despite considerable medical resistance to these findings.

Could it be that the same great advances in technology that—in the hands of controlled biomedical science—have markedly reduced disease, might—in the hands of the food industry—cause an equally marked but unrecognized nutritional disease? In particular, could they cause a lipid-centered malnutrition that could account for the modernization-disease group, and for the fact that life expectancy in the mid-years of the human life span increased so little during the 100 years between 1850 and 1950, even though we have conquered the major killers of 100 years ago?

Such questions led me to evaluate the national dietary consumption figures and to compare them with disease incidences. The results show that modern food processing and food selection processes severely distort the availability of many essential nutrient and antinutrient families—especially by limiting the Omega-3 essential fatty acids—and that, wherever this occurs, the incidence of modernization diseases skyrockets. In fact, heart disease and certain cancers are finally being recognized as primarily linked to distortions of dietary fats. But what is most discouraging is that the heart and cancer experts rarely refer to one another's findings.

Why? Because this would make their two pet illnesses—heretofore considered unrelated—merely symptomatic variations of a single underlying nutritional disorder, the modernization-disease syndrome. Nutritionists and biochemists have overlooked this new illness syndrome because they think mainly in terms of single nutrient effects and single illnesses, now divided among a multitude of medical specialties. They have forgotten how clinically variable nutritional disorders, such as beriberi and pellagra, can be. Finally, the unique dependence of humans on the Omega-3 essential fatty acids explains why the usual nutritional laboratory work on nonprimates has been misleading.

Nutritional synergism exists between most of the components of our diet. For example, the essential fatty acids are protected from destruction in the body by the antioxidants, consisting of vitamins, A, C, and E, and selenium and beta-carotene. In turn, the essential fatty acids are converted by the B vitamins into the fat-based regulatory system, including the prostaglandins, which regulate almost every bodily function at the tissue level. This nutritional synergism and the extensiveness of the regulatory systems affected by nutrition explain why, although no single food modification is responsible, a large number of small food modifications affecting different essential nutrients and antinutrients can interact to cause many different illnesses, depending on genetic susceptibility. It also explains why the therapeutic efficacy of all contemporary diets can be significantly enhanced by adding to them the nutritional missing link—the Omega-3 essential fatty acids. Because of this missing link, the full power of nutritional supplementation therapy—our primary line of treatment, or orthopharmacology—has not been realized until now, with the result that we too quickly turn to the therapeutic drugs of the physician—our secondary pharmacology.

Nutritional synergism also answers many of the major concerns of medicine and nutrition today. It explains why megadosing can be beneficial, at least for a while. It explains why so many different schools of nutrition claim similar benefits. For example, it explains why elevated serum cholesterol has been shown to be lowered by supplements of fiber alone, niacin alone, or Omega-3 fats alone, and why all three taken together, in combination with removal of saturated fat and other antinutrients, will produce the greatest benefit. It explains why B vitamins and Omega-3 fatty acids supplements can separately correct various skin disorders. Similarly, it explains how, starting in the early 1950s, three different reform nutrition groups could correctly claim that dietary problems underlie our major illnesses.

T. L. Cleave and the British fiber theorists have provided strong evidence that a dietary fiber deficiency in modernized societies contributes to a variety of bowel and bowel-related illnesses, such as peptic ulcer, gallstones, irritable bowel syndrome (spastic colon or mucous colitis), diverticulitis, diabetes, and elevated serum fats. Other British researchers—H. M. Sinclair, J. Reed, and others—have provided evidence that an Omega-3 deficiency is related to elevated serum-cholesterol levels and cardiovascular diseases, including heart attacks, angina pectoris, and strokes, each of which is also a modernization disease.

Abram Hoffer of Victoria, B.C. has noted that our modern disease picture, ranging from schizophrenia to many physical illnesses, looks a great deal like old-fashioned B-vitamin deficiency pellagra, except that it is vitamin resistant—a "Hoffer pellagra." For this reason, Hoffer has been a major force behind the introduction of megavitamin therapy, while at the same time urging a return to the consumption of nonprocessed, natural foods, the goal being to achieve a diet approximating the traditional human diet. The traditional diet, compared with our contemporary diet, contains vastly greater amounts of essential nutrients, including dietary fiber, Omega-3 fatty acids, selenium, and many B vitamins—as well as far lesser amounts of the antinutrients, including saturated fat, "funny fats" (the isomers produced by hydrogenation), and sugar.

The fiber supplements recommended by Cleave, the Omega-3 essential fatty acid supplements recommended by Sinclair and Reed, and the niacin supplements recommended by Hoffer each reduce elevated serum fats when taken separately. I show in this book that, especially when taken together and combined with a lowered intake of antinutrients, they ameliorate many other modernization diseases as well. Clearly, supplementation programs must include both Omega-6 and Omega-3 fats, and vitamin and mineral antioxidants (including vitamins C and E, selenium, cysteine, and beta-carotene), as well as work toward a reduction of antinutrient toxicity effects produced by excessive consumption of saturated fat, sugar, salt, and "funny fats." In brief, we must return to the traditional natural diet if we are to prevent, ameliorate, and cure the modernization-disease syndrome and its associated accelerated aging disease.

In my opinion, the current universal medical teaching asserting that scientists in the United States, Holland, and Japan (Goldberger, Eijkmann, and Takaki) solved the problem of beriberi and pellagra around the turn of the century is wrong. What they solved was the B-vitamin deficiency form of these problems, while leaving unidentified the much broader fat-centered deficiency-toxicity form that accounts for the bulk of disease today in modernized societies. In my opinion, the medical profession has been misdiagnosing and mistreating the bulk of its cases for fifty to a hundred years or more.

The Omega-3 essential fatty acids family—the cold-climate ultrapolyunsaturates that come mainly from northern plants and fish—turn out to be the essential nutrient especially required by humans. They are also the unique factor in the cod-liver oil supplements of our youth. Consequently, the facts recounted in this book can be viewed as reintroducing and scientifically updating the old-fashioned cod-liver oil regimen. This is accomplished by using high Omega-3 foods and purified supplements, including flaxseed oil, which are appropriate for temperate and cold climates, in particular using these as therapeutic supplements for short periods of time in conjunction with antioxidants and other cofactors in the treatment of overt illness.

In support of this line of reasoning, I conducted a new kind of clinical pilot study in forty-four patient volunteers over a period of several years. This study followed each case intensively over two to three years and, at the same time, cut across virtually the entire spectrum of medical specialties, both physical and mental. Consequently, what

I am presenting here is not the usual statistical study of large numbers of patients all belonging to a single symptomatic disease group and studied by one specialty or another. Rather, it is an entirely new kind of individually intensive cross-specialty diagnostic and therapeutic investigation.

The study used supplements of food-grade flaxseed oil, a high Omega-3 oil from plant sources. Flaxseed oil (also known as linseed oil) can be viewed as an approximate alternative to cod-liver oil and other fish oils. However, only plant oils such as flaxseed oil contain alpha linolenic acid (ALA), which alone manipulates certain body enzymes. The fish oils lack this essential fatty acid but contain higher Omega-3 essential fatty acids, which manipulate other related enzymes. As a result, the plant and fish Omega-3 fatty acids can have different therapeutic effects, as I discuss in this book.

So that spontaneous remission and placebo effects could be excluded, I accepted cases for study only if the individuals had long-term chronic illness that had failed to respond adequately to extensive orthodox medical treatment. In addition, the patients were mostly professionals who did not fit the placebo-reactor personality profile. I also often cycled the patients off and on the flaxseed oil supplement or substituted low Omega-3 oils (safflower or corn) and found that improvement varied accordingly. Double blinds were impractical in this pilot study, especially since taste differences in the oils are marked. Finally, once improvement was seen with the oils, the other dietary corrections and vitamin supplements noted above were introduced if the patients were not already on them as part of their previous treatment, which was left untouched.

The clinical results can only be called spectacular. In addition to ameliorating many specific modern illnesses, both physical and mental, the findings also indicate that stamina, vigor, and feelings of mental equanimity and well-being can be restored to many people who have been underperforming for many years, often without fully realizing it. Other reform nutritionists who have informally evaluated the regimen in their own practices for one to two years tell me they are seeing similar major benefits. Of course, formal confirmatory trials are needed. Nevertheless, the implications are clear, and I would consider it imprudent not to make the findings public at this point.

Some subjects report further improvement as the result of adding evening primrose oil, a relatively highly unsaturated form of the Omega-6 essential fatty acids. The goal is to correct the basic diet and, when needed, to fine-tune the ratio of the oils used as supplements to fit each person's specific nutritional needs. Just as a single nutritional distortion can induce a variety of illnesses in different people because of differences in genetic susceptibility, so people can have varying requirements for nutritional supplements, especially if they are ill. In some cases, improvement can be seen within hours or, more often, weeks. Other benefits take four to six months. Of course, severe cases may have suffered irreversible damage, in which case they cannot respond at all.

Some evidence indicated that doses tolerated in colder climates, say Philadelphia in winter, can become overdoses on taking a winter vacation in, say Mexico, causing such things as muscular aches and excessive lassitude. This is consistent with the fact that the Omega-3 oils are produced rather specifically in response to a cold climate, the more fluid Omega-3 helping to protect cell membranes from the effects of congealing. Thus, in cold climates more Omega-3 is normally produced by the food chain and consumed by humans, while less is produced and perhaps needed in warmer climes. But requirements may depend on genetic type independent of the ambient climate.

The patients in my study were encouraged to slowly self-titrate the dose up or down—for example, increasing or decreasing by 50 percent per week—and to be careful to avoid excess, since this can cause a flare-up of the original problems even after remission has been produced at lower dosages. Since the patients were all chronic cases who had not responded to a variety of other treatments, the placebo effect was not a major concern. But Omega-6 supplements served to test the specificity of the effects, although as indicated, double-blind studies were not practical because of the distinctive flavor of the different oils.

These are important matters. The evidence indicates that our modern lifestyle diseases are our primary public health hazard, costing us more than any world war and now putting our society at risk in many unrecognized ways, extraclinical and social as well as clinical. Conversely, intelligent action can bring rewards exceeding those resulting from Pasteur's discovery of the cause of infectious disease and from Goldberger's discovery of the cause of classical pellagra as a B-vitamin deficiency disease.

I think that modern nutritional deficiencies may account for over half of all disease. But I also think there are—and have seen—wonderful cures and vigorous good health when adequate nutrition, through supplements and diet, is part of a healthy lifestyle.

REFERENCES

Preface

Rudin DO. "The Dominant Diseases of Modernized Societies as Omega-3 Essential Fatty Acid Deficiency Syndrome: Substrate Beriberi." *Medical Hypotheses* 8:17, 1982.

Rudin DO. "The Major Psychoses and Neuroses as Omega-3 Essential Fatty Acid Deficiency Syndrome: Substrate Pellagra." *Biological Psychiatry* 16:837, 1981.

Rudin DO and Felix C, with Schrader C. *The Omega-3 Phenomenon: The Nutritional Breakthrough of the '80s.* New York: Rawson Associates, 1987.

Chapter 1
The Missing Nutrient

Bogert LJ, Briggs GM, and Calloway DH. *Nutrition and Physical Fitness.* Ninth Edition. Philadelphia: W.B. Saunders Company, 1973.

Carpenter KJ, ed. *Pellagra.* Benchmark Papers in Biochemistry, Vol. 2. Stroudsburg, PA: Hutchinson Ross Publishing Company, 1981.

Fiennes RN, Sinclair AJ, and Crawford MA. "Essential Fatty Acid Studies in Primates: Linolenic Acid Requirements of Capuchins." *Journal of Medical Primatology* 2:155, 1973.

Rudin DO. "The Dominant Diseases of Modernized Societies as Omega-3 Essential Fatty Acid Deficiency Syndrome: Substrate Beriberi." *Medical Hypotheses* 8:17, 1982.

Rudin DO. "The Major Psychoses and Neuroses as Omega-3 Essential Fatty Acid Deficiency Syndrome: Substrate Pellagra." *Biological Psychiatry* 16:837, 1981.

Rudin DO and Felix C, with Schrader C. *The Omega-3 Phenomenon: The Nutritional Breakthrough of the '80s.* New York: Rawson Associates, 1987.

Shils ME, Olson JA, and Shike M, eds. *Modern Nutrition in Health and Disease.* Eighth Edition. Philadelphia: Lea & Febiger, 1994.

Chapter 2
Some Fats Are Good for You

Bracco U and Deckelbaum R, eds. *Polyunsaturated Fatty Acids in Human Nutrition.* Nestlé Nutrition Workshop Series, Vol. 28. New York: Raven Press, 1992.

Cunnane SC and Thompson LU, eds. *Flaxseed in Human Nutrition.*

Champaign, IL: AOCS Press, 1995.

Galli C and Simopoulos A, eds. *Dietary Omega-3 and Omega-6 Fatty Acids*. New York and London: Plenum Press, 1989.

Hattersley J. "Lowering Cholesterol with Lovastatin, The Wrong Approach: A Survey of Usually Overlooked Literature." *Journal of Orthomolecular Medicine* 9:54, 1994.

Horrobin DF. *The Prostaglandins: Physiology, Pharmacology and Clinical Aspects*. St. Albans, VT: Eden Medical Research, 1978.

Jacobs D, Blackburn H, and others. "Report on the Conference on Low Blood Cholesterol: Mortality Associations." *Circulation* 86: 1046, 1992.

Kolata G. "Cholesterol's New Image: High is Bad; So Is Low." *The New York Times*, 11 August 1992.

Lands WEM. *Polyunsaturated Fatty Acids and Eicosanoids*. Champaign, IL: AOCS Press, 1987.

Leaf A and Weber P. "A New Era for Science in Nutrition." *The American Journal of Clinical Nutrition* 45(supplement):1048, 1987.

Neaton J, Blackburn H, and others. "Serum Cholesterol Level and Mortality Finding for Men Screened in the Multi-Risk Factor Intervention Trial." *The Archives of Internal Medicine* 152:1490, 1992.

Rudin DO and Felix C, with Schrader C. *The Omega-3 Phenomenon: The Nutritional Breakthrough of the '80s*. New York: Rawson Associates, 1987.

Scientific Review Committee. *Nutrition Recommendations*. Report H49-42/1990E. Ottawa: Minister of National Health and Welfare, 1990.

Simopoulos AP. "Omega-3 Fatty Acids in Health and Disease and In Growth and Development." *The American Journal of Clinical Nutrition* 54:438–463, 1991.

Sinclair A and Gibson R, eds. *Essential Fatty Acids and Eicosanoids*. Invited papers from the Third International Congress. Champaign, IL: AOCS Press, 1992.

Sinclair HM. "Essential Fatty Acids in Perspective." *Human Nutrition: Clinical Nutrition* 38C:245, 1984.

Chapter 3
Our Deteriorating Diet

Burkett D. *Eat Right—To Keep Healthy and Enjoy Life More*. New York: Arco, 1979.

Cade JF. "The Aetiology of Schizophrenia." *Medical Journal of Australia* 2:135, 1956.

Carpenter DL and Slover HT. "Lipid Composition of Selected Margarines." *Journal of the American Oil Chemists' Society* 50:372, 1973.

Cleave TL. *The Saccharine Disease:*

The Master Disease of Our Time.
New Canaan, CT: Keats, 1975.

Dohan FD. "Schizophrenia: Are
some food derived polypeptides
pathogenic? Celiac disease as a
model." In *The Biological Basis of
Schizophrenia,* G Hemmings and
WA Hemmings, eds. MTP Press,
1979.

Eaton SB, Shostak M, and Konner
M. *The Paleolithic Prescription.*
New York: Harper & Row, 1988.

Fiennes RN, Sinclair AJ, and
Crawford MA. "Essential Fatty
Acid Studies in Primates: Li-
nolenic Acid Requirements of
Capuchins." *Journal of Medical Pri-
matology* 2:155, 1973.

Flower RJ and Blackwell GJ.
"Anti-inflammatory Steroids Induce Biosynthesis of a Phospholi-
pase A2 Inhibitor Which Prevents
Prostaglandin Synthesis." *Nature*
278:456, 1979.

Goodhart RS and Shils ME. *Modern Nutrition in Health and Disease.*
Philadelphia: Lea & Febiger, 1973.

Holman, RT. "A Long Scaly
Tale—The Study of Essential
Fatty Acid Deficiency at the University of Minnesota." In *Essential
Fatty Acids and Eicosanoids,* A Sinclair and R Gibson, eds. Champaign, IL: AOCS Press, 1992.

Holman RT and others. "A Case of
Human Linolenic Acid Deficiency
Involving Neurological Abnor-
malities." *The American Journal of
Clinical Nutrition* 35:617, 1982.

Kinsella JE and others. "Metabolism of Trans Fatty Acids." *The
American Journal of Clinical Nutrition* 34:2307, 1981.

Kirschman JD. *Nutrition Almanac.*
New York: McGraw-Hill, 1979.

Kramsch DM and others. "Reduction of Coronary Artery Atherosclerosis by Moderate Condition-
ing Exercise in Monkeys on an
Atherogenic Diet." *New England
Journal of Medicine* 305:1483, 1981.

Lamptey MS and Walker BL. "A
Possible Essential Role for Dietary
Linolenic Acid in the Development
of the Young Rat." *Journal of Nutrition* 106:86, 1976.

Owren PA. "Coronary Thrombosis: Its Mechanism and Possible
Prevention by Linolenic Acid."
Annals of Internal Medicine 63:167,
1965.

Page LB and others. "Antecedents of Cardiovascular Disease
in Six Solomon Islands Societies."
Circulation 49:1132, 1974.

Rudin DO. "The Major Psychoses
and Neuroses as Omega-3 Essential Fatty Acid Deficiency Syndrome: Substrate Pellagra." *Biological Psychiatry* 16:837, 1981.

Torrey EF. *Schizophrenia and Civi-
lization.* Northvale, NJ: Jason
Aronson, 1980.

Trowell HC. *Noninfective Diseases
in Africa.* London: Arnold, 1960.

Trowell HC and Burkitt DP. *West-*

ern Diseases: Their Emergence and Prevention. Cambridge, MA: Harvard University Press, 1981.

Trowell HC, Burkitt DP, and Heaton D, eds. *Dietary Fibre, Fibre-Depleted Foods and Disease.* New York: Academic Press, 1985.

United States Department of Commerce. *Historical Statistics of the U.S.: Colonial Times to 1970.* Washington, DC: Bureau of the Census, 1975.

Chapter 4
How the Omega Program Developed—The Forty-Four-Patient Study
Rudin DO. "The Dominant Diseases of Modernized Societies as Omega-3 Essential Fatty Acid Deficiency Syndrome: Substrate Beriberi." *Medical Hypotheses* 8:17, 1982.

Rudin DO. "The Major Psychoses and Neuroses as Omega-3 Essential Fatty Acid Deficiency Syndrome: Substrate Pellagra." *Biological Psychiatry* 16:837, 1981.

Rudin DO and Felix C, with Schrader C. *The Omega-3 Phenomenon: The Nutritional Breakthrough of the '80s.* New York: Rawson Associates, 1987.

Chapter 5
Ridding Ourselves of Modern-Day Plagues
Abeywardena MY, McLennan PL, and Charnock JS. "Role of

Eicosanoids in Dietary Fat Modification of Cardiac Arrhythmia and Ventricular Fibrillation." In *Essential Fatty Acids and Eicosanoids,* A Sinclair and R Gibson, eds. Champaign, IL: AOCS Press, 1992.

Anderson JW and others. "Health Benefits and Practical Aspects of High-Fiber Diets." *American Journal of Clinical Nutrition* 59(supplement):1242-S, 1994.

Bailey C. *Fit or Fat?* Boston: Houghton Mifflin Co., 1977.

Bang HO, Dyerberg J, and Brondum Nielsen A. "Plasma Lipids and Lipoprotein Pattern in Greenlandic West Coast Eskimos." *The Lancet* 1:1143, 1971.

Belluzzi A, Brignola C, and others. "Effect of an Enteric-coated Fish-oil Preparation on Relapses in Crohn's Disease." *The New England Journal of Medicine* 334:1557, 1996.

Billman GE, Hallaq H, and Leaf A. "Prevention of Ischemia-induced Ventricular Fibrillation by Omega 3 Fatty Acids." *Proceedings of the National Academy of Science U.S.A.* 91:4427, 1994.

Borkman M and others. "The Relation Between Insulin Sensitivity and the Fatty-Acid Composition of Skeletal-Muscle Phospholipids." *The New England Journal of Medicine* 328:238, 1993.

Bracco U and Deckelbaum RJ, eds.

Polyunsaturated Fatty Acids in Human Nutrition. Nestlé Nutrition Workshop Series, Vol. 28. New York: Raven Press, Ltd., 1992.

Charnock JS. "Dietary Fats and Cardiac Arrhythmia in Primates." *Nutrition* 10:161, 1994.

Cohen LA and others. "Effect of Varying Proportions of Dietary Menhaden and Corn Oil on Experimental Rat Mammary Tumor Promotion." *Lipids* 28:449, 1993.

Cunnane SC. "Metabolism and Function of Alpha-linolenic Acid in Humans." In *Flaxseed in Human Nutrition*, SC Cunnane and LU Thompson, eds. Champaign, IL: AOCS Press, 1995.

de Lorgeril M and others. "Mediterranean Alpha Linolenic Acid-Rich Diet in Secondary Prevention of Coronary Heart Disease." *The Lancet* 343:1454, 1994.

Hattersley J. "Lowering Cholesterol with Lovastatin, The Wrong Approach: A Survey of Usually Overlooked Literature." *Journal of Orthomolecular Medicine* 9:54, 1994.

Horrobin DF. "Nutritional and Medical Importance of Gamma-Linolenic Acid." *Progress in Lipid Research* 31:163–194, 1992.

Jacobs D, Blackburn H, and others. "Report on the Conference on Low Blood Cholesterol: Mortality Associations." *Circulation* 86:1046, 1992.

Jamal GA and Carmichael H. "Gamma-Linolenic Acid in Diabetic Neuropathy." *Diabetic Medicine* 75:319, 1990.

Jialal I and Grundy SM. "Effect of Dietary Supplementation with Alpha Tocopherol on the Oxidative Modification of Low Density Lipoprotein." *Journal of Lipid Research* 33:899, 1992.

Karmali RA and others. "Plant and Marine Omega-3 Fatty Acids Inhibit Experimental Metastasis of Rat Mammary Adenocarcinoma Cells." *Prostaglandins, Leukotrienes, and Essential Fatty Acids* 48:309, 1993.

Klehm TG and others. "Beneficial Effects of High Fiber Diet in Hyperglycemic Diabetic Men." *American Journal of Clinical Nutrition* 29:895, 1976.

Kolata G. "Cholesterol's New Image: High is Bad; So Is Low." *The New York Times*, 11 August 1992.

Kurzer MS, Slavin JL, and Adlercreutz H. "Flaxseed, Lignans, and Sex Hormones." In *Flaxseed in Human Nutrition*, SC Cunnane and LU Thompson, eds. Champaign, IL: AOCS Press, 1995.

Leaf A and Weber PC. "Medical Progress: Cardiovascular Effects of Omega-3 Fatty Acids." *The New England Journal of Medicine* 318:549–557, 1988.

Lees RS and Karel M, eds. *Omega-3 Fatty Acids in Health and Disease.*

New York and Basel: Marcel Dekker, Inc., 1990.

Neaton J, Blackburn H, and others. "Serum Cholesterol Levels and Mortality Finding for Men Screened in the Multi-Risk Factor Intervention Trial." *The Archives of Internal Medicine* 152:1490, 1992.

Nettleton JA. "Are Omega-3 Fatty Acids Essential Nutrients for Fetal and Infant Development?" *Journal of the American Dietetic Association* 93:58, 1993.

Okuyama H. "Effects of Dietary Essential Fatty Acid Balance on Behavior and Chronic Disease." In *Polyunsaturated Fatty Acids in Human Nutrition*, U Bracco and RJ Deckelbaum, eds. Nestlé Nutrition Workshop Series, Vol. 28. New York: Raven Press, Ltd., 1992.

Owren PA. "Coronary Thrombosis: Its Mechanism and Possible Prevention by Linolenic Acid." *Annals of Internal Medicine* 63:167, 1965.

Rifici VA and Khachadurian AK. "Oxidation of High Density Lipoprotein: Characteristics and Effects on Cholesterol Efflux From J774 Macrophages." *Biochimica et Biophysica Acta* 1299:87, 1996.

Rivellese A and others. "Effect of Dietary Fiber on Glucose Control and Serum Lipoproteins in Diabetic Patients." *The Lancet* 2:447, 1980.

Setchell KDR. "Discovery and Potential Clinical Importance of Mammalian Lignans." In *Flaxseed in Human Nutrition*, SC Cunnane and LU Thompson, eds. Champaign, IL: AOCS Press, 1995.

Setchell KDR and Adlercreutz H. "Mammalian Lignans and Phytooestrogens. Recent studies on Their Formation, Metabolism and Biological Role in Health and Disease." In *Role of the Gut Flora in Toxicity and Cancer*, I Rowland, ed. London: Academic Press, 1988.

Simopoulos AP. "Omega-3 Fatty Acids in Health and Disease and In Growth and Development." *The American Journal of Clinical Nutrition* 54:438–463, 1991.

Sinclair HM. "Prevention of Coronary Heart Disease: The Role of Essential Fatty Acids." *Postgraduate Medical Journal* 56:579, 1980.

Stenson WF and others. "Dietary Supplementation with Fish Oil in Ulcerative Colitis." *Annals of Internal Medicine* 116:609–614, 1992.

Stephens NG and others. "Randomised controlled trial of vitamin E in patients with coronary disease: Cambridge Heart Antioxidant Study (CHAOS)." *The Lancet* 347:781, 1996.

Stubbs CD. "The Structure and Function of Docosahexaenoic Acid in Membranes." In *Essential Fatty Acids and Eicosanoids*. Champaign, IL: AOCS Press, 1992.

Tamura Y and others. "Anti-Atherogenic and Anti-Inflammatory Action of Omega-3 Polyunsaturated Fatty Acids." In *Essential Fatty Acids and Eicosanoids,* A Sinclair and R Gibson, eds. Champaign, IL: AOCS Press, 1992.

Thompson LU. "Flaxseed, Lignans, and Cancer." In *Flaxseed in Human Nutrition,* SC Cunnane and LU Thompson, eds. Champaign, IL: AOCS Press, 1995.

Tisdale MJ. "Essential Fatty Acids and Cancer." In *Essential Fatty Acids and Eicosanoids,* A Sinclair and R Gibson, eds. Champaign, IL: AOCS Press, 1992.

Watkins TR and others. "Improving Atherogenic Risk Factors with Flaxseed Bread." *Proceedings of the 55th Flax Institute of the United States.* Fargo, North Dakota, 1994.

Chapter 6
The Omega Complexion Connection
Bagchi K and others. "The Etiology of Phrynoderma." *American Journal of Clinical Nutrition* 7:251, 1958.

Holman RT. "Significance of Essential Fatty Acids in Human Nutrition." *Lipids* 1:215, 1976.

Holman RT. "Biological Activities of and Requirements for Polyunsaturated Acids." *Progress in the Chemistry of Fats and Other Lipids* 9:607–682, 1970.

Munnich A and others. "Fatty Acid Responsive Alopecia in Multiple Carboxylase Deficiency." *The Lancet* 1:1080, 1980.

Rudin DO. "The Dominant Diseases of Modernized Societies as Omega-3 Essential Fatty Acid Deficiency Syndrome: Substrate Beriberi." *Medical Hypotheses* 8:17, 1982.

Rudin DO. "The Major Psychoses and Neuroses as Omega-3 Essential Fatty Acid Deficiency Syndrome: Substrate Pellagra." *Biological Psychiatry* 16:837, 1981.

Rudin DO and Felix C, with Schrader C. *The Omega-3 Phenomenon: The Nutritional Breakthrough of the '80s.* New York: Rawson Associates, 1987.

Shils ME, Olson JA, and Shike M, eds. *Modern Nutrition in Health and Disease.* Eighth Edition. Philadelphia: Lea & Febiger, 1994.

Chapter 7
Omega Nutrition and Reproductive Health
Auger J and others. "Decline in Semen Quality Among Fertile Men in Paris During the Past 20 Years." *New England Journal of Medicine* 332:281, 1995.

Burr GO and Burr MM. "On the Nature and Role of the Fatty Acids Essential in Nutrition." *Journal of Biological Chemistry* 86:587, 1929.

Crawford M and Marsh D. *Nutrition and Evolution.* New Canaan, CT: Keats Publishing, Inc., 1995.

Galli C, Trzeciak HI, and Paoletti R. "Effects of Dietary Fatty Acids on the Fatty Acid Composition of Brain Ethanolamine Phosphoglyceride." *Biochimica et Biophysica Acta* 248:449, 1971.

Hardy A. "Was Man More Aquatic in the Past?" *The New Scientist* 7:642, 1960.

Jeremy JY. "Long Chain Fatty Acids in Obstetrics, Gynecology, and Fertility." In *Polyunsaturated Fatty Acids in Human Nutrition*, U Bracco and R Deckelbaum, eds. Nestlé Nutrition Workshop Series, Vol. 28. New York: Raven Press, Ltd., 1992.

"Male Reproductive Health and Environmental Oestrogens." *The Lancet* 345:933, 1995.

Monique DM and others. "Essential Fatty Acids, Pregnancy and ʾPregnancy Outcome." Abstract in Fatty Acids and Lipids From Cell Biology to Human Disease. Second International Congress of the ISS-FAL International Society for the Study of Fatty Acids and Lipids, June, 1995.

Nettleton JA. "Are Omega-3 Fatty Acids Essential Nutrients for Fetal and Infant Development?" *Journal of the American Dietetic Association* 93:58, 1993.

Price WA. *Nutrition and Physical Degeneration*. La Mesa, CA: Price-Pottenger Nutrition Foundation, 1945.

Quackenbush FW, Kummerow FA, and Steenbock HJ. "The Effectiveness of Linoleic, Arachidonic and Linolenic Acids in Reproduction and Lactation." *Journal of Nutrition* 24:213, 1943.

Rudin DO and Felix C, with Schrader C. *The Omega-3 Phenomenon: The Nutritional Breakthrough of the '80s*. New York: Rawson Associates, 1987.

Skakkebaek NE and Keiding N. "Changes in Semen and the Testis." *British Medical Journal* 309: 1316, 1994.

Svennerholm L. "Distribution and Fatty Acid Composition of Phosphoglycerides in Normal Human Brain." *Journal of Lipid Research* 9:570, 1968.

Vallette G and others. "Dynamic Pattern of Estradiol Binding to Uterine Receptors of the Rat. Inhibition and Stimulation by Unsaturated Fatty Acids." *Journal of Biological Chemistry* 263:3639, 1988.

Chapter 8
The Omega-Strong Infant and Toddler

Benson JD and others. "Modifications of Lipids in Infant Formulas: Concerns of Industry." In *Essential Fatty Acids and Eicosanoids*, A Sinclair and R Gibson, eds. Champaign, IL: AOCS Press, 1992.

Carlson SE. "The Role of PUFA in Infant Nutrition." *Inform* 6:940, 1995.

Colquhoun I and Bunday S. "A

Lack of Essential Fatty Acids as a Possible Cause of Hyperactivity in Children." *Medical Hypotheses* 7:673, 1981.

Connor WE, Neuringer M, and Lin DS. "Dietary Effects on Brain Fatty Acid Composition: The Reversibility of Omega-3 Fatty Acid Deficiency and Turnover of Docosahexaenoic Acid in the Brain, Erythrocytes, and Plasma of Rhesus Monkeys." *Journal of Lipid Research* 31:237, 1990.

Crawford M and Marsh D. *Nutrition and Evolution.* New Canaan, CT: Keats Publishing, Inc, 1995.

Eaton SB, Shostak M, and Konner M. *The Paleolithic Prescription.* New York: Harper & Row, 1988.

Enig MG. "Fats and Oils: Understanding the Functions and Properties of Partially Hydrogenated Fats and Oils and Their Relationship to Unhydrogenated Fats and Oils." *Townsend Letter for Doctors* 125:1212, 1993.

Holman RT. "A Long Scaly Tale—The Study of Essential Fatty Acid Deficiency at the University of Minnesota." In *Essential Fatty Acids and Eicosanoids*, A Sinclair and R Gibson, eds. Champaign, IL: AOCS Press, 1992.

Horrobin DF. "Nutritional and Medical Importance of Gamma-Linolenic Acid." *Progress in Lipid Research* 31:163–194, 1992.

Kaplan BJ, McNicol J, and others.

"Dietary Replacement in Preschool-Aged Hyperactive Boys." *Pediatrics* 83:7, 1989.

Kinney HC and others. "Decreased Muscarinic Receptor Binding in the Arcuate Nucleus in Sudden Infant Death Syndrome." *Science* 269:1446, 1995.

Kneebone GM, Kneebone R, and Gibson RA. "Fatty Acid Composition of Breast Milk From Three Racial Groups From Penang, Malaysia." *The American Journal of Clinical Nutrition* 41:765, 1985.

Koletzko B. "Long-chain Polyunsaturated Fatty Acids in Infant Formulae in Europe." *ISSFAL (International Society for the Study of Fatty Acids and Lipids) Newsletter* 2:3, 1995.

Mannuzza S, Klein R, and others. "Hyperactive Boys Almost Grown Up, V—Replication of Psychiatric Status." *Archives of General Psychiatry* 48:77, 1991.

Martineau J and others. "Effects of Vitamin B-6 on Averaged Evoked Potentials in Infantile Autism." *Biological Psychiatry* 16:625, 1981.

Mitchell EA, Aman MG, and others. "Clinical Characteristics and Serum Essential Fatty Acid Levels in Hyperactive Children." *Clinical Pediatrics* 26:406, 1987.

Price WA. *Nutrition and Physical Degeneration.* La Mesa, CA: Price-Pottenger Nutrition Foundation, 1945.

Rimland B, Callaway E, and Dreyfus P. "The Effects of High Doses of Vitamin B6 on Autistic Children: A Double-Blind Crossover Study." *American Journal of Psychiatry* 135:472, 1978.

Rudin DO. "The Dominant Diseases of Modernized Societies as Omega-3 Essential Fatty Acid Deficiency Syndrome: Substrate Beriberi." *Medical Hypotheses* 8:17, 1982.

Rudin DO. "The Major Psychoses and Neuroses as Omega-3 Essential Fatty Acid Deficiency Syndrome: Substrate Pellagra." *Biological Psychiatry* 16:837, 1981.

Rudin DO and Felix C, with Schrader C. *The Omega-3 Phenomenon: The Nutritional Breakthrough of the '80s.* New York: Rawson Associates, 1987.

Salmon MB. *Breast Milk—Nature's Perfect Formula.* Techkits, Inc., P.O. Box 105, Demarest NJ, 1994.

Shils ME, Olson JA, and Shike M, eds. *Modern Nutrition in Health and Disease.* Eighth Edition. Philadelphia: Lea & Febiger, 1994.

Stevens, LJ, Zentall S, and others. "Essential Fatty Acid Metabolism in Boys with Attention-Deficit Disorder." *The American Journal of Clinical Nutrition* 62:761, 1995.

Todd RD and Ciaranello RD. "Demonstration of Inter- and Intra-Species Differences in Serotonin Binding Sites by Antibodies From an Autistic Child." *Proceedings of the National Academy of Sciences of the U.S.A.* 82:612, 1985.

Yonekubo A, Honda S, and others. "Physiological Role of Docosahexaenoic Acid in Mother's Milk and Infant Formula." In *Essential Fatty Acids and Eicosanoids,* A Sinclair and R Gibson, eds. Champaign, IL: AOCS Press, 1992.

Chapter 9
The Omega Way to Mental Health

Abdullah YH and Hamadah K. "Effect of ADP on PGE Formation in Blood Platelets from Patients with Depression, Mania and Schizophrenia." *British Journal of Psychiatry* 127:591, 1975.

Adams R. "Approach to Patients with Neurological and Psychiatric Disease.0 In *Harrison's Principles of Internal Medicine.* Seventh Edition. New York: McGraw-Hill, 1974.

Erin D. "The Missing Nutritional Link That Cured My Ten Years of Schizophrenia." *Alternative Medicine Digest* 7:10–13, 1995.

Hoffer A. "Chronic Schizophrenic Patients Treated Ten Years or More." *Journal of Orthomolecular Medicine* 8:7–37, 1993.

Hoffer A. *Common Questions on Schizophrenia and Their Answers.* New Canaan, CT: Keats Publishing, Inc., 1987.

Hoffer A and Osmond H. "Treatment of Schizophrenia With Nicotinic Acid—A Ten Year Followup." *Acta Psychiatrica Scandinavica* 40:171, 1964.

Horrobin DF, ed. *Omega-6 Essential Fatty Acids: Pathophysiology and Roles in Clinical Medicine.* New York: Alan Liss, 1990.

Olds ME. "Hypothalamic Substrate for the Positive Reinforcing Properties of Morphine in the Rat." *Brain Research* 168:351, 1979.

Rudin DO. "The Dominant Diseases of Modernized Societies as Omega-3 Essential Fatty Acid Deficiency Syndrome: Substrate Beriberi." *Medical Hypotheses* 8:17, 1982.

Rudin DO. "The Major Psychoses and Neuroses as Omega-3 Essential Fatty Acid Deficiency Syndrome: Substrate Pellagra." *Biological Psychiatry* 16:837, 1981.

Rudin DO and Felix C, with Schrader C. *The Omega-3 Phenomenon: The Nutritional Breakthrough of the '80s.* New York: Rawson Associates, 1987.

Shils ME, Olson JA, and Shike M, eds. *Modern Nutrition in Health and Disease.* Eighth Edition. Philadelphia: Lea & Febiger, 1994.

Chapter 10
The Omega Antiaging Diet
Ausman LM and Russell RM. "Nutrition in the Elderly." In *Modern Nutrition in Health and Disease,* ME Shils, JA Olson, and J Shike, eds. Eighth Edition. Philadelphia: Lea & Febiger, 1994.

Gershon D and others. "Characterization and Possible Effects of Age-Associated Alterations in Enzymes and Proteins." *Aging* 8:21, 1979.

Hall DA and Burdett PE. "Age Changes in Metabolism of Essential Fatty Acids." *Biochemical Society Transactions* 3:42, 1975.

Hart RW and Setlow RB. "Correlation Between DNA Excision Repair and Lifespan in a Number of Mammalian Species." *Proceedings of the National Academy of Sciences* 71:2169, 1974.

Hayflick L. "The Cell Biology of Human Aging." *Scientific American* 242:58, 1980.

Horrobin DF. "Loss of Delta-6-Desaturase Activity as a Key Factor in Aging." *Medical Hypotheses* 7:1211, 1981.

Kraemer KH. "Progressive Degenerative Diseases Associated with Defective DNA Repair Process." In *DNA Repair Processes, Cellular Senescence, and Somatic Cell Genetics,* WW Nichols and DG Murphy, eds. Year Book Medical, 1979.

Prickett JD and others. "Dietary Enrichment with Polyunsaturated Fatty Acid Eicosapentaenoic Acid Prevents Proteinuria and Prolongs Survival in NZB X NZW F1 Mice." *Journal of Clinical Investigation* 68:556, 1981.

Chapter 11
The Omega Program—Phases 1 and 2
Enig MG. "Trans Fatty Acids—An

Update." Research review. *Nutrition Quarterly* 17:79–95, 1993.

Food and Nutrition Board, National Research Council. *Recommended Dietary Allowances*. Tenth Edition. Washington, DC: National Academy Press, 1989.

Koletzko B. "Trans Fatty Acids May Impair Biosynthesis of Long-Chain Polyunsaturates and Growth in Man." *Acta Paediatrica* 81:302, 1992.

Mensink RP and Katan MB. "Effect of Dietary Trans Fatty Acids on High-Density and Low-Density Lipoprotein Cholesterol Levels in Healthy Subjects." *New England Journal of Medicine* 323:439, 1990.

Shils ME, Olson JA, and Shike M. *Modern Nutrition in Health and Disease*. Eighth Edition. Philadelphia: Lea & Febiger, 1994.

Stephens NG and others. 8Randomised controlled trial of vitamin E in patients with coronary disease: Cambridge Heart Antioxidant Study (CHAOS)." *The Lancet* 347:781, 1996.

Chapter 12
The Omega Program—Phases 3 and 4

Horrobin DF. "Nutritional and Medical Importance of Gamma-Linolenic Acid." *Progress in Lipid Research* 31:163–194, 1992.

Jamal GA and Carmichael H. "Gamma-Linolenic Acid in Diabetic Neuropathy." *Diabetic Medicine* 75:319, 1990.

Kunin RA. *Meganutrition: The New Prescription for Maximum Health, Energy and Longevity*. New York: New American Library, 1981.

Appendix A
Sources of Omega Fatty Acids

Anderson BA. "Comprehensive Evaluation of Fatty Acids in Foods. VII. Pork Products." *Journal of the American Dietetic Association* 69:44, 1976.

Anderson BA and others. "Comprehensive Evaluation of Fatty Acids in Foods. II. Beef Products." *Journal of the American Dietetic Association* 67:67, 1975.

Anderson BA and others. "Comprehensive Evaluation of Fatty Acids in Foods. X. Lamb and Veal." *Journal of the American Dietetic Association* 70:53, 1977.

Bitman J and others. "Comparison of the Lipid Composition of Breast Milk from Mothers of Term and Preterm Infants." *American Journal of Clinical Nutrition* 38:300, 1983.

Brignoli CA, Kinsella JE, and Weihrauch JL. "Comprehensive Evaluation of Fatty Acids in Foods. V. Unhydrogenated Fats and Oils." *Journal of the American Dietetic Association* 68:224, 1976.

Gibson RA and Kneebone GM. "Fatty Acid Composition of Human Colostrum and Mature Breast Milk." *American Journal of Clinical Nutrition* 34:252, 1981.

Guthrie HA and others. "Fatty Acid Pattern of Human Milk." *Journal of Pediatrics* 90:39, 1977.

Exler J and Weihrauch JL. "Comprehensive Evaluation of Fatty Acids in Foods. VIII. Finfish." *Journal of the American Dietetic Association* 69:243, 1976.

Exler J and Weihrauch JL. "Comprehensive Evaluation of Fatty Acids in Foods. XII. Shellfish." *Journal of the American Dietetic Association* 71:518, 1977.

Exler J and others. "Comprehensive Evaluation of Fatty Acids in Foods. XI. Leguminous Seeds." *Journal of the American Dietetic Association* 71:412, 1977.

Fristrom GA and Weihrauch JL. "Comprehensive Evaluation of Fatty Acids in Foods. IX. Fowl." *Journal of the American Dietetic Association* 69:517, 1976.

Fristrom GA and others. "Comprehensive Evaluation of Fatty Acids in Foods. IV. Nuts, Peanuts, and Soups." *Journal of the American Dietetic Association* 67:351, 1975.

Hepburn FN, Exler J, and Weihrauch JL. "Provisional Tables on the Content of Omega-3 Fatty Acids and Other Fat Components of Selected Foods." *Journal of the American Dietetic Association* 86:788, 1986.

James WPT and Theander O, eds. *The Analysis of Dietary Fiber in Food.* New York and Basel: Marcel Dekker, Inc., 1981.

Kneebone GM, Kneebone R, and Gibson RA. "Fatty Acid Composition of Breast Milk from Three Racial Groups from Penang, Malaysia." *American Journal of Clinical Nutrition* 41:765, 1985.

Lanza E and Butrum RR. "A Critical Review of Food Fiber Analysis and Data." *Journal of the American Dietetic Association* 86:732, 1986.

Posati LP, Kinsella JE, and Watt BK. "Comprehensive Evaluation of Fatty Acids in Foods. I. Dairy Products." *Journal of the American Dietetic Association* 66:482, 1975.

Posati LP and others. "Comprehensive Evaluation of Fatty Acids in Foods. III. Eggs and Egg Products." *Journal of the American Dietetic Association* 67:111, 1975.

Simopoulos AP and Salem Jr. N. "Egg Yolk as a Source of Long-chain Polyunsaturated Fatty Acids in Infant Feeding." *American Journal of Clinical Nutrition* 55:11, 1992.

Weiss ES and Wolfson RP. *Cholesterol Counter.* New York: Jove Publications, 1973.

Appendix B
A Note to Physicians

Bogert LJ, Briggs GM, and Calloway DH. *Nutrition and Physical Fitness.* Ninth Edition. Philadelphia: W.B. Saunders Company, 1973.

Burkett, D. *Eat Right—To Keep*

Healthy and Enjoy Life More. New York: Arco, 1979.

Carpenter DL and Slover HT. "Lipid Composition of Selected Margarines." *Journal of the American Oil Chemists' Society* 50:372, 1973.

Carpenter KJ, ed. *Pellagra.* Benchmark Papers in Biochemistry, Vol. 2. Stroudsburg, PA: Hutchinson Ross Publishing Co., 1981.

Cleave TL. *The Saccharine Disease: The Master Disease of Our Time.* New Canaan, CT: Keats, 1975.

Goodhart RS and Shils ME. *Modern Nutrition in Health and Disease.* Philadelphia: Lea & Febiger, 1973.

Hoffer, A. "Chronic Schizophrenic Patients Treated Ten Years or More." *Journal of Orthomolecular Medicine* 8:7–37, 1993.

Hoffer A and Osmond H. "Treatment of Schizophrenia with Nicotinic Acid—A Ten Year Followup." *Acta Psychiatrica Scandinavica* 40:171, 1964.

Kirschman JD. *Nutrition Almanac.* New York: McGraw-Hill, 1979.

National Food Survey Committee. *Household Food Consumption and Expenditure: 1973.* London: Her Majesty's Stationery Office, 1974.

Page LB and others. "Antecedents of Cardiovascular Disease in Six Solomon Islands Societies." *Circulation* 49:1132, 1974.

Reed SA. "Dietary Source of Omega-3 Eicosapentaenoic Acid." *The Lancet* 2:739, 1979.

Rudin DO. "The Dominant Diseases of Modernized Societies as Omega-3 Essential Fatty Acid Deficiency Syndrome: Substrate Beriberi." *Medical Hypotheses* 8:17, 1982.

Rudin DO. "The Major Psychoses and Neuroses as Omega-3 Essential Fatty Acid Deficiency Syndrome: Substrate Pellagra." *Biological Psychiatry* 16:837, 1981.

Rudin DO and Felix C, with Schrader C. *The Omega-3 Phenomenon: The Nutritional Breakthrough of the '80s.* New York: Rawson Associates, 1987.

Sinclair HM. "Prevention of Coronary Heart Disease: The Role of Essential Fatty Acids." *Postgraduate Medical Journal* 56:579, 1980.

Trowell HC. *Noninfective Diseases in Africa.* London: Arnold, 1960.

Trowell HC and Burkitt DP. *Western Diseases: Their Emergence and Prevention.* Cambridge, MA: Harvard University Press, 1981.

United States Department of Commerce. *Historical Statistics of the U.S.: Colonial Times to 1970.* Washington, DC: Bureau of the Census, 1975.

GLOSSARY

Italicized words are defined elsewhere in the Glossary.

Adipose cells. The scientific term for cells that contain the body's fat stores.

Alpha linolenic acid (ALA). The primary member of the *Omega-3* family of *essential fatty acids*. The body converts ALA into either *docosahexaenoic acid* or *eicosapentaenoic acid*. ALA is found in high quantities in flaxseed oil.

Angina pectoris. Acute chest pain caused by spasms that squeeze the coronary arteries.

Antinutrient. A substance, such as white flour, refined sugar, or *trans-fatty acid*, that hinders the actions of nutrients. The modern diet contains a high amount of antinutrients.

Antioxidant. Any of a large group of substances whose presence slows down the deterioration of *fatty acids* caused by oxygen and other substances. Antioxidants include vitamins C and E, the vitamin A precursor beta-carotene, and the mineral selenium.

Arachidonic acid (ARA). A member of the *Omega-6* family of *essential fatty acids*. The body makes ARA from the primary Omega-6, *linoleic acid*.

Arrhythmia. A disturbance of the heartbeat. An arrhythmia can be fatal, and can occur in persons with no history of cardiovascular disease.

Atherosclerosis. The buildup of fatty deposits, known as plaques, in the arteries. Atherosclerosis can lead to a heart attack or stroke if the affected artery becomes completely blocked.

Attention-deficit hyperactivity disorder (ADHD). A term used to describe children who are disruptively inattentive, impulsive, and hyperactive.

Beriberi. A disease, caused by a B-vitamin deficiency, with symptoms that range from nerve degeneration to fluid retention.

Cholesterol. A complex fatty substance that performs a variety of tasks within the body. Cholesterol cannot move through the bloodstream by itself, but must be packaged into either *high-density lipoprotein* or *low-density lipoprotein* before it can circulate throughout the body.

Cold pressed. Oil that has been extracted by putting mechanical pressure on batches of seeds without the use of heat.

Docosahexaenoic acid (DHA). A member of the *Omega-3* family of *essential fatty acids.* The body makes DHA from the primary Omega-3, *alpha linolenic acid.* DHA is found in high quantities in cold-water fish and marine animals.

Double bond. A place in the carbon chain of a *fatty acid* where hydrogen atoms have been removed. The more double bonds a fatty acid has, the more fluid the fat will be.

Eczema. A general term that refers to itching and inflamed, scaling, and oozing skin.

Eicosanoids. Chemicals created by the body to regulate a wide variety of processes. The eicosanoids include the *prostaglandins.*

Eicosapentaenoic acid (EPA). A member of the *Omega-3* family of *essential fatty acids.* The body makes EPA from the primary

Omega-3, *alpha linolenic acid*. EPA is found in high quantities in cold-water fish and marine animals.

Enzyme. A protein produced by the body to facilitate a chemical reaction, but which itself is unchanged by the reaction.

Essential fatty acid (EFA). A *fatty acid* that the body cannot manufacture by itself, but which must be supplied in the diet. There are two families of EFAs, the *Omega-3* fats and the *Omega-6* fats.

Fatty acid. A chain of carbon atoms that has an acid attached to one end, with hydrogen atoms attached to the rest of the carbon atoms in the chain.

Fiber. Any of several indigestible substances that form the "roughage" of plant material. Fiber aids in bowel regularity, helps to stabilize blood sugar, and aids in the elimination of *cholesterol* from the body.

Free radical. A molecule or a piece of a molecule with a single, or unpaired, electron. Since it is seeking to be paired, this molecule steals electrons from other electron pairs. Although free radical reactions generally occur in normal bodily processes, they can pose a danger when they are involved in an uncontrolled chain reaction.

Gamma linolenic acid (GLA). A member of the *Omega-6* family of *essential fatty acids*. The body makes GLA from the primary Omega-6, *linoleic acid*. GLA can sometimes mimic and augment the effects of *Omega-3* fatty acids within the body, and is found in high quantities in evening primrose oil.

High-density lipoprotein (HDL). A substance that carries fats and *cholesterol* through the bloodstream. It consists of cholesterol combined with an *essential fatty acid* surrounded by protein. HDL is thought to be the "good" substance that returns excess cholesterol to the liver.

Hydrogenation. A commercial process that solidifies oils by saturating the *double bonds* in *fatty acids* with hydrogen. This process produces a number of artificial substances, including *trans-fatty acids*.

Irritable bowel syndrome (IBS). A digestive-system condition marked by abdominal pain, gas, and diarrhea. It is also known as spastic colon or mucous colitis.

Lignan. A plant fiber that becomes special mammalian lignan when acted upon by the intestines' natural bacteria. It has been shown to have antitumor effects in humans. Flaxseed is the richest available source.

Lignin. A plant fiber related to cellulose that, together with cellulose, forms the woody cell walls of plants. It is one component of dietary *fiber*.

Linoleic acid. The primary member of the *Omega-6* family of essential fatty acids. The body converts linoleic acid into *arachidonic acid* and *gamma linolenic acid*.

Low-density lipoprotein (LDL). A substance that carries fats and *cholesterol* through the bloodstream. It consists of cholesterol combined with an *essential fatty acid* surrounded by protein. LDL is thought to be the "bad" substance that deposits cholesterol along the artery walls, although there is evidence that this only occurs when LDL becomes *oxidized*.

Manic-depressive disorder. A mental disorder characterized by either deep depression or alternating periods of depression and mania.

Modernization-disease syndrome. A group of diseases and conditions, including *atherosclerosis,* cancer, *irritable bowel syndrome, schizophrenia,* and *eczema,* that is linked to the nutritional distortions of the modern diet. These disorders include both the presence of numerous *antinutrients* and the absence of many important nutrients, including various *antioxidants* and the *Omega-3* oils.

Monounsaturated. A *fatty acid* that contains one *double bond* between carbon atoms in its chain.

Nonessential fatty acid (NEFA). A *fatty acid* that the body can manufacture by itself.

Omega-3. A family of *essential fatty acids;* the primary Omega-3 is *alpha linolenic acid.* The modern diet generally supplies very little Omega-3.

Omega-6. A family of *essential fatty acids;* the primary Omega-6 is *linoleic acid.* The modern diet generally has much more Omega-6 than *Omega-3,* thus creating an imbalance.

Osteoarthritis. A form of arthritis caused by wear and tear on the joints.

Oxidation. The addition of oxygen, subtraction of hydrogen, or addition of electrons to a substance. Oxidation is usually accompanied by a release of energy. It is also the process by which fats become rancid.

Pellagra. A disease, caused by a B-vitamin deficiency, with symptoms that include skin problems, dementia, digestive problems, fatigue, and headache.

Polyunsaturated. A *fatty acid* that contains more than one *double bond* between carbon atoms in its chain. Polyunsaturates can be either *regular polyunsaturates* or *ultrapolyunsaturates.*

Premenstrual syndrome (PMS). A group of symptoms experienced before the start of the menstrual period that includes nervous tension, breast tenderness, fatigue, headache, and food cravings.

Prostaglandin. A substance, created from an *essential fatty acid,* that regulates many different bodily processes, including functioning of the cardiovascular, digestive, reproductive, and nervous systems. Each essential fatty acid produces its own prostaglandin.

Regular polyunsaturates. Another term for the *Omega-6* oils. It refers to the fact that these oils have more hydrogen atoms, and are thus less fluid, than the *ultrapolyunsaturates.*

Rheumatoid arthritis. A form of arthritis in which the immune system attacks the joints.

Saturated fatty acid. A *fatty acid* with no *double bonds* within its carbon chain—the chain is completely saturated by hydrogen. Saturated fats are solid at room temperature.

Schizophrenia. A mental disorder characterized by hallucinations, delusions, and detachment from reality.

Seborrheic dermatitis. A skin condition characterized by dandruff of the eyebrows and red, patchy skin around the eyes, nose, or cheeks, or on the outer ear canals.

Sudden infant death syndrome (SIDS). A condition in which infants die without warning from unknown causes. It is also called crib death.

Trans-fatty acids. Artificial *fatty acids* produced by *hydrogenation*. These imposter fatty acids displace, and hinder the work of, natural fatty acids.

Ultrapolyunsaturates. Another term for the *Omega-3* oils. It refers to the fact that these oils have fewer hydrogen atoms, and are thus more fluid, than the *regular polyunsaturates*.

ABOUT THE AUTHORS

Donald O. Rudin, MD, attended the University of Colorado and then received his medical degree from Harvard Medical School in 1948. He went into basic research, and the work he and his colleagues did on the nerve impulse in cells resulted in a patent.

In 1956, Dr. Rudin became the founding director of the Department of Molecular Biology at the Eastern Pennsylvania Psychiatric Institute in Philadelphia, on the recommendation of the Rockefeller Institute's Nobelist director, Herbert Gasser. There, Dr. Rudin and his colleagues did research on cell membranes and nerve impulses, research that led Dr. Rudin to see a link between the Omega-3 essential fatty acids and dietary deficiencies caused by modern food refining processes, a problem he called the modernization-disease syndrome.

Dr. Rudin then worked to explore cell theory in connection with the brain and how it processes knowledge. He has written about his efforts in this area in *Axiomatic Epistemology and World Theory.*

Dr. Rudin has sat on fund-granting agencies and has numerous publications to his credit.

Clara Felix took as her role model the biochemist Adelle Davis, who wrote that eating the right foods could prevent the diseases caused by dietary deficiencies. In response to Davis's work, Ms. Felix used her four children and the family dog as nutritional guinea pigs, and enrolled in the University of California at Berkeley after her children were grown, where she received her B.S. in nutrition science. In 1981, she began publishing *The Felix Letter: A Commentary on Nutrition.* Inquiries about her bimonthly newsletter can be addressed to her at P.O. Box 7094, Berlekey CA 94707.

INDEX

Acne, effect of flaxseed oil on,
   76–77
ADHD. *See* Attention-deficit
   hyperactivity disorder.
Aging
   "death gene" and, 128–129,
      130, 134
   diseases associated with,
      128
   enzyme production and,
      128–129, 130, 131
   genetics and, 128–130
   "immortality gene" and,
      128–129, 134
   prostaglandins and, 129
   ways to fight process of,
      132–134
Agoraphobia, 111
   effect of flaxseed oil on,
      115–117
ALA. *See* Alpha linolenic acid.
Allergies, food, testing for,
   153–156
Alopecia areata, effect of
   flaxseed oil on, 75

Alpha linolenic acid (ALA), 14,
   16
   diabetes and, 64
   heart disease and, 57–58
   response to Omega Program
      and, 159
   sources of, 22–23
Angina pectoris, 54
   effect of flaxseed oil on, 42
Antinutrients
   action of, in body, 37
   as factor leading to disease,
      37
   in average American diet, 7
   increased consumption of,
      27–28
   reduction of, and Omega
      Program, 142
Antioxidants
   aging and, 131, 133
   deficiency of, as factor leading
      to disease, 36
   Omega Program and, 148
   oxidation of cholesterol and,
      53

See also Beta-carotene; Selenium; Vitamin A; Vitamin C; Vitamin E.
Anxiety attacks, 110–111
ARA. *See* Arachidonic acid.
Arachidonic acid (ARA), 14
    brain and, 88, 102
    in breast milk, 102
Arrhythmias, effect of Omega-3 on, 54–55
Atherosclerosis, 52. *See also* Heart attacks.
Attention-deficit hyperactivity disorder (ADHD), 97–98
Autism, 98–99

B vitamins
    deficiency of, and skin problems, 78–79
    deficiency of, as cause of disease, 3–5, 35
    megadoses of, 145
    mental illness and, 114, 118
    Omega Program and, 144–145
    reduced consumption of, 27
    sources of, 145
    See also Niacin; Thiamin.
Benign prostatic hypertrophy.
    See Enlarged prostate.
Beriberi, 3
Beta-carotene, 36, 143, 144
Blood clots
    as cause of heart attacks, 53–54
    prostaglandins and, 54
Breastfeeding, benefits of, 100–103, 104
Burkitt, Denis, 2, 33

Calcium, 147. *See also* Minerals.
Cancer
    aging and, 134
    fiber and, 33, 61
    genetic damage and, 129
    mammalian lignan and, 61

nutrition and, 60–61
    traditional Japanese diet and, 25–26
Cardiovascular problems, effect of flaxseed oil on, 42–43, 58.
    See also Heart attacks.
Children, Omega Program and.
    See Breastfeeding, benefits of; Toddlers, proper diet for.
Cholesterol
    and antioxidants, 53
    conversion of, into lipoprotein, 17
    functions of, 15, 17, 71
    heart disease and, 52–53, 55
    importance of, for infants, 101
    reduction of, and fiber, 33
    reduction of, and health problems, 18
    sources of, 13
Chronic intestinal inflammation, effect of fish oil on, 67–68
Cleave, T. L., 2, 33
Crawford, Michael, 90
Crohn's disease, effect of fish oil on, 67

Davis, Adelle, 2
"Death gene," 128–129, 130, 134
Dental problems, 91, 99–100
DHA. *See* Docosahexaenoic acid.
Diabetes
    deficiency of essential fatty acids and, 63
    fiber and, 64
Diet, modern
    aging and, 131
    autism and, 99
    beriberi and, 3
    dental problems and, 91, 99–100
    disease and, 2, 7, 9, 23–24, 25–27, 28–29, 91
    hydrogenation and, 30–31

increased consumption of beef
in, 30
Norwegian notch, 26–27
nutrient depletion in, 5, 21, 24,
27–28
pellagra and, 4–5
pregnant women and, 89–91
reduction of whole grains in,
30
See also Antinutrients.
Discoid lupus, effect of flaxseed
oil on, 77–78
Disease, factors leading to, 34–37
Docosahexaenoic acid (DHA), 14
attention-deficit hyperactivity
disorder (ADHD) and, 97–98
brain and, 88, 102
diabetes and, 64
in breast milk, 102
in infant formula, 103–104
male sexual health and, 86
sources of, 22
vision and, 64, 108

Eczema, effect of flaxseed oil on,
78. *See also* Skin problems.
Eicosanoids, 18. *See also*
Prostaglandins.
Eicosapentaenoic acid (EPA), 14
aging and, 131
sources of, 22
Emotional problems
effect of flaxseed oil on, 43
modernization-disease
syndrome and, 111
See also Agoraphobia; Anxiety
attacks; Manic-depressive
disorder; Paranoia;
Schizophrenia.
Enlarged prostate, 86–87
Enzymes
conversion of Omega fats and,
142
production of, and aging,
128–131

EPA. *See* Eicosapentaenoic acid.
Essential fatty acids, 6–8
aging and, 129–131
cholesterol and, 17
diabetes and, 63–64
disorders caused by
deficiencies of, 6–7
female infertility and, 84–85
fetal brain development and,
88–89
mental illness and, 112
pregnancy and, 88–92
skin and, 71–72
types of, 14
vaginal dryness and, 85
See also Omega-3 fatty acids;
Omega-6 fatty acids.
Exercise
aging and, 133
benefits of, 36–37
Omega Program and, 161

Fat, 12. *See also* Monounsaturated fat; Polyunsaturated
fat; Saturated fat; Unsaturated fat.
Fatty acids
composition of, 12
role of, in body, 6
See also Essential fatty acids;
Nonessential fatty acids.
Fiber
aging and, 133
cancer prevention and, 33,
61–62
cholesterol reduction and, 33
deficiency of, as factor leading
to disease, 36
importance of, for toddlers,
107
insulin production and, 32–33,
64
Omega Program and, 149–150
recommended daily intake of,
33–34

reduced consumption of, 27
role of, in body, 32
types of, 32
Fish oil
  as source of Omega-3 fatty
    acids, 5
  balancing with flaxseed oil,
    163–164
  effect of, on attention-deficit
    hyperactivity disorder
    (ADHD), 98
  effect of, on heart disease, 56,
    60
  effect of, on intestinal
    problems, 67–68
  in Eskimo traditional diet, 59
  pregnancy and, 23, 89
  reduction of thromboxane
    and, 56
  See also Alpha linolenic acid;
    Docosahexaenoic acid;
    Eicosapentaenoic acid.
Flaxseed oil
  as source of Omega-3 fatty
    acids, 5
  balancing with other oils, 160,
    163–165
  buying and storing, 137–138
  correct dosage of, 139–140
  effect of, on acne, 76–77
  effect of, on agoraphobia,
    115–117
  effect of, on alopecia areata,
    75
  effect of, on angina pectoris,
    42
  effect of, on discoid lupus,
    77–78
  effect of, on eczema, 78
  effect of, on emotional
    problems, 43
  effect of, on enlarged prostate,
    87
  effect of, on headaches,
    43–44
  effect of, on high blood
    pressure, 42
  effect of, on immune
    disorders, 44–45
  effect of, on manic-depressive
    disorder, 118–120
  effect of, on menopause,
    46–47
  effect of, on menstrual
    irregularity, 82
  effect of, on phrynoderma,
    75–76
  effect of, on Raynaud's
    disease, 44
  effect of, on rheumatoid
    arthritis, 45
  effect of, on schizophrenia,
    120–123
  effect of, on urinary tract
    problems, 47–48
  miscellaneous benefits of, 48
  Omega Program and,
    136–140
  possible side effects of, 160,
    162–163
  pregnancy and, 23
  production of lignan and, 62
  See also Alpha linolenic acid.
Food Damage Report, 27–28
Forty-four patient study, 5–6,
    39–49
  enlarged prostate and, 87
  female infertility and, 84–85
  menstrual irregularity and, 82
  mental illness and, 114–123
  skin problems and, 73–78

Galli, C., 88
Gamma linolenic acid (GLA)
  attention-deficit hyperactivity
    disorder (ADHD) and, 98
  diabetes and, 64
  evening primrose oil and, 64,
    165
  infant formula and, 103, 104

Genetics
    aging and, 128–130
    as factor leading to disease,
      34–35
    mental illness and, 113
    progeria and, 129–130
    xeroderma pigmentosa and,
      129–130
GLA. *See* Gamma linolenic acid.

Hair loss, sudden. *See* Alopecia
    areata.
Hardy, Sir Alister, 90
Headaches, effect of flaxseed oil
    on, 43–44
HDL. *See* High-density lipo-
    protein.
Heart attacks
    atherosclerosis as cause of,
      51–52
    blood clots and, 53–54
    conditions leading to, 53
    lack of fiber and, 33
    saturated fat and, 31
    See also Cardiovascular
      problems.
High blood pressure, effect of
    flaxseed oil on, 42
High-density lipoprotein (HDL),
    17
    deficiency of, and heart
      attacks, 53
    oxidation of, and athero-
      sclerosis, 52
    See also Cholesterol.
Hoffer, Abram, 2, 124
Holman, Ralph T., 7
Horrobin, David, 64
Hydrogenation, 13
    production of trans-fatty acids
      and, 31
    to combat rancidity, 30–31

IBS. *See* Irritable bowel
    syndrome.

"Immortality gene," 128–129, 134
Immune disorders
    effect of flaxseed oil on, 44–45
    lack of Omega-3 fatty acids
      and, 66
Infant formula, 103–105
    vegetarian supplements and,
      106
Infertility
    female, essential fatty acids
      and, 84–85
    male, effect of DDT on, 86
    male, essential fatty acids and,
      86
Intermittent claudication, 56
    effect of flaxseed oil on, 42–43
Intestinal problems, effect of fish
    oil on, 67–68
Irritable bowel syndrome (IBS),
    relief of, on Omega Program,
    45–46

LDL. *See* Low-density lipo-
    protein.
Linoleic acid, 14, 16, 89
Lipoproteins
    Lipoprotein (a), role of, in
      heart disease, 57
    See also High-density lipo-
      protein; Low-density lipo-
      protein.
Low-density lipoprotein (LDL),
    17
    excess of, and heart attacks,
      53
    oxidation of, and athero-
      sclerosis, 52
    See also Cholesterol.

Malnutrition, aging and, 131–132
Mammalian lignan
    as deterrent to cancer, 61
    production of, by flaxseed, 62
Manic-depressive disorder, 110,
    117

effect of flaxseed oil on,
118–120
Meganutrients, excessive intake
of, 141–142
Menopause, effect of flaxseed oil
on, 46–47
Menstrual cramps, 83–84
Menstrual irregularity, effect of
flaxseed oil on, 82
Minerals
deficiency of, as factor leading
to disease, 35–36
loss of, in food processing, 27
See also Calcium; Selenium;
Trace minerals; Zinc.
Modernization-disease
syndrome
attention-deficit hyperactivity
disorder (ADHD) and, 97
effects of Omega Program on,
49
mental illness and, 111
Monounsaturated fat, 13

Neurospora, 134
Niacin (vitamin B₃)
cholesterol levels and, 33
pellagra and, 4–5
See also B vitamins.
Nonessential fatty acids, 6, 14
Norwegian notch, 26–27

Obesity
health problems associated
with, 65
overcoming, 66
Okuyama, Harumi, 66
Omega Program, 8, 10, 39–49,
135–166
antioxidants and, 148
average response times to,
158
B vitamins and, 144–145
calcium and, 147
cofactors of, 140–149

effect of, on mental illness,
114–125
effect of, on sex drive, 86
effect of, on skin conditions,
73–80
fiber and, 149
finding optimum level of, 157,
159–160
irritable bowel syndrome and,
45–46
miscellaneous benefits of, 48
osteoarthritis and, 46
pilot study of, 39–49
selenium and, 148
treatment involved in, 41
vitamin A and, 143–144
vitamin C and, 145–146
vitamin E and, 146
Omega-3 fatty acids
aging and, 130, 132
balance of cholesterol and, 18
deficiency of, and mental
illness, 111–114
deficiency of, and sudden
infant death syndrome
(SIDS), 96–97
deficiency of, and skin, 71–72
deficiency of, as factor leading
to disease, 35
diabetes and, 64
difference between Omega-6
fatty acids and, 14
effect of, on blood, 56–57
eicosanoids and, 18
importance of, to health, 15
menstrual cramps and, 84
premenstrual syndrome
(PMS) and, 83
production of, and climate,
14–15
recommended daily intake of,
22
reduced consumption of, 23,
27
sources of, 5, 22, 136

See also Alpha linolenic acid;
Docosahexaenoic acid;
Eicosapentaenoic acid.
Omega-6 fatty acids
balancing with flaxseed oil,
164–165
diabetes and, 64
difference between Omega-3
fatty acids and, 14
eicosanoids and, 18
importance of, to health, 15
menstrual cramps and, 84
production of, and climate,
14–15
recommended daily intake of,
22
sources of, 38
See also Arachidonic acid;
Gamma linolenic acid;
Linoleic acid.
Osmond, Humphrey, 124
Osteoarthritis, relief of, on
Omega Program, 46

Paranoia, 111
Pauling, Linus, 124
Pellagra, 3–5
Phrynoderma, effect of flaxseed
oil on, 75–76
PMS. *See* Premenstrual
syndrome.
Polyunsaturated fat, 13, 16
Pregnancy
essential fatty acids and,
88–92
proper nutrition and, 91–92
Premenstrual syndrome (PMS),
82–83
Price, Florence, 91
Price, Weston A., 89, 91, 99–100
Progeria, 129–130
Prostacyclin, 54
Prostaglandins
aging and, 129–131
blood clotting and, 54

bodily functions affected by,
19
function of, 20
headaches and, 43–44
heart rhythm and, 54–55
hormones and, 19, 63, 83
imbalance of, and health
problems, 20–21
imbalance of, and mental
illness, 112, 114
menstrual cramps and, 83–84
premenstrual syndrome
(PMS) and, 83
rheumatoid arthritis and, 45
skin and, 71–72
vitamin B_6 and, 144
Pro-vitamin A. *See* Beta-carotene.

Raynaud's disease, effects of
flaxseed oil on, 44
Rheumatoid arthritis, effects of
flaxseed oil on, 45

Saturated fat
composition of, 12
heart attacks and, 31
increased consumption of, 28
Schizophrenia, 111
effect of flaxseed oil on,
120–123
Selenium
importance of taking, with
flaxseed oil, 162
Omega Program and, 148
reduced consumption of, 27
See also Minerals.
SIDS. *See* Sudden infant death
syndrome.
Sinclair, H. M., 2
Skin
as indicator of health, 152, 157
composition of, 70–71
essential fatty acids and, 71–72
function of, 70–71
vitamin A and, 143

See also Skin problems.
Skin problems
    effect of flaxseed oil on, 47,
        73–80
    effect of Omega Program on,
        152, 157
Stenson, William, 68
Stress
    as factor leading to disease,
        36
    reducing, and Omega
        Program, 161
Sudden infant death syndrome
    (SIDS), 96–97
Svennerholm, Lars, 88

Thiamin (vitamin B₁), 3. *See also*
    B vitamins.
Thromboxane
    arrhythmia and, 54–55
    excess of, and atherosclerosis,
        54
    reduction of, and fish oil, 56
Toddlers, proper diet for,
    105–107
Trace minerals, 148–149
Trans-fatty acids, 13
    action of, on body, 31
    attention-deficit hyperactivity
        disorder (ADHD) and, 98
    creation of, by hydrogenation,
        31

Ulcerative colitis, effect of fish
    oil on, 67–68

Unsaturated fat
    blood-cholesterol level and,
        17, 31
    composition of, 12–13
    types of, 13
    See also Monounsaturated fat;
        Polyunsaturated fat.
Urinary tract problems
    effect of flaxseed oil on, 47–48

Vaginal dryness, essential fatty
    acids and, 85. *See also*
    Menopause, effect of flax-
    seed oil on.
Varicose veins, effect of flaxseed
    oil on, 42–43
Vitamin A, Omega Program
    and, 143–144. *See also*
    Antioxidants.
Vitamin B. *See* B vitamins.
Vitamin C
    deficiency of, and athero-
        sclerosis, 57
    in toddler diet, 106–107
    Omega Program and,
        145–146
    sources of, 146
    See also Antioxidants.
Vitamin E, Omega Program and,
    146. *See also* Antioxidants.

Xeroderma pigmentosa, 129–130

Zinc, skin problems and, 78–79.
    See also Minerals.